D1550378

Prescriptions For Healthy Farm Animals

By Dr. John B. Herrick

A Farmer's Digest Publication, Brookfield, Wis.

Publisher's Cataloging in Publication
(Prepared by Quality Books Inc.)

Herrick, John B., 1919-
   Prescriptions for healthy farm animals / John B. Herrick. --
   p. cm.
   ISBN 0-944079-01-6

   1. Animal health. 2. Livestock--Diseases. 3. Veterinary public
health.   I. Title.

SF65.2   636.08

                                  90-92107
                                     MARC

International Standard Book
Number: 0-944079-01-6.

Library of Congress Catalog
Card Number: 90-92107.

Published by Farmer's Digest Books, A Division of
   No-Till Farmer, Inc.
P.O. Box 624, Brookfield, Wisconsin 53008-0624.
Manufactured in the United States of America.

Production Editor: Kelly Lessiter
Cover Design: Laura Plank

A Few Words About This Practical Book...

IF YOU ARE an animal owner, you certainly have a responsibility to provide your animals with the best of management and care.

Just like humans, animals suffer pain if given rations which are deficient in either quality or quantity. Animals that suffer from parasitism and various ailments not only suffer pain, but do not respond well when productivity is measured.

A healthy animal utilizes feed more efficiently, grows faster, produces a better quality product and reaches the market quicker than a sick or diseased animal. More than ever before, animal owners are also concerned about their animals' welfare.

This book is designed to help you raise healthy livestock by developing a thorough understanding of animal health. It will show you how to spot the signs and symptoms of disease and to determine when veterinary assistance is needed. This book is not a substitute for veterinary assistance, but, hopefully, its pages will provide you with the information necessary to determine when to call a veterinarian before costly losses occur.

Each day more consumers of meat, milk and eggs are asking for animal protein which is of the highest quality and free from drug residues. It is your responsibility to provide such products—a producer who does not will jeopardize all other products, just like one bad apple in a barrel. Therefore, emphasis must be placed on the judicious use of drugs and biologics in the production of all animals. Never before have animal owners been saddled with such grave responsibility and trust.

The information in this book is based on research findings along with a generous dose of "first hand knowledge." You'll also find many "tricks of the trade" that you can use.

This manual is plastic-bound for daily use in the barn or pasture. Written especially for farmers who want to stop costly losses from unnecessary animal death and disease, cut costs and have healthier, more profitable livestock, its easy-to-understand directions and step-by-step illustrations show you how to prevent losses, detect diseases in early stages and do many preliminary jobs which will save the veterinarian's valuable time. This book is not meant to replace your veterinarian, but to supplement his efforts and help you market more livestock at the lowest possible cost.

A benefit you can receive from frequent use of this book is the ability to always be conscious of your animals' state of health. This book will help you recognize trouble before it really strikes and to avoid the crippling losses which can wreck your livestock enterprise.

Since the prevention of diseases and parasites is much more economical than relying upon treatment, this book places greater emphasis on prevention instead of treatment. A comfortable animal is less apt to become diseased, therefore all animal production should be programmed so genetics, nutrition, environment and management are interrelated with accurate health records which can serve as valuable guidlines. Remember that animal production without health records is like driving a car without brakes or a steering wheel.

—Dr. John Herrick

Livestock Record Sheets Go Hand-In-Hand With This Book!

To make this book's information more valuable, you need good animal health and management records.

AS YOU PAGE through this book, you'll find the author strongly recommends that you keep individual health and management records on all of your animals.

It Really Pays Off! All this information can help you and your veterinarian do a much better job of managing and treating problem animals. This essential information will go a long way toward improving the health and profitability of your farm animals.

There's no easier way to gather this information than by using the Livestock Production And Health Record Sheets shown in detail on the following pages in this book:

Beef Cattle—157 and 158.
Dairy Cattle—215 and 216.
Sow/Litter—284 and 285.

Ewe/Lamb—335 and 337.

Easy To Use! Available in sets of 100 forms each, these Record Sheets will let you keep full details on the health and management practices used with all of your animals. A three-ring loose-leaf binder is also available for properly safe-keeping your Record Sheets.

Keeping good records is certainly essential for healthy farm animals and these sheets can make your record-keeping duties fast and easy.

For further details and prices on the four types of Livestock Production And Health Record Sheets and/or the handy three-ring loose-leaf binder, contact: Farmer's Digest Library, P.O. Box 624, Brookfield, Wisconsin 53008-0624.

Table Of Contents

General Health Practices

Cattle

Beef Cattle

Dairy Cattle

Swine

Sheep

Goats

Horses

Poultry

References

Chapter 1

Your Responsibilities As An Animal Owner

NO ONE SHOULD own animals of any type or number unless they can provide adequate care and facilities. Furthermore, you should recognize the needs of animals in the area of nutrition along with those factors necessary to prevent disease.

Animals need "preventive maintenance" from you in the form of vaccines, parasite control and other key factors which are essential to keep your animals comfortable and growing efficiently. The best approach is to put together a health program—a prearranged calendarized set of practices for the maintenance of health from your veterinarian—and then follow it carefully. Through the Cooperative Extension Service, each state also has such programs available for all species of animals.

The next important factor, particularly with horses and cattle, is to provide adequate handling facilities. Animals need to be restrained so they can be vaccinated, dewormed and treated for injuries. Properly constructed corrals, chutes, and stanchions are a necessity for safe, humane handling of animals.

The following guidelines are necessary to identify and to render proper first aid to animals:

1 Know the animals' behavior and their habits. Animals who are off feed often have an abnormal gait and stance or rapid respiration, diarrhea, and physical appearance that should be easily spotted. This means seeing and observing animals daily or as frequently as possible.

Animals attempting to give birth should be observed even more frequently. If in labor for more than 1 to 2 hours, they should have the attendance of a veterinarian. This points out the need for essential records for all animals so critical periods of the animal's life can be properly recorded.

2 Don't excite or stress an apparently sick animal. Death is frequently hastened by attempting to restrain or move the animal.

3 Record temperatures, length of time the animal has been "down" or ill and report this to your veterinarian. Observe animals both in the early morning and again in the afternoon so your veterinarian can determine if it is an emergency that requires his immediate attention.

4 Try to be on hand when the veterinarian arrives. There is nothing more disconcerting than for a veterinarian to try to find, restrain and treat an animal without the presence of the owner. In no case should a child be left to aid in the control of an unruly or aggressive sick animal. Have ample warm water, light and restraint for the animal already available when the veterinarian arrives.

5 Some animals will die and they should be disposed of immediately. Rendering services should be called immediately for large animals. Burial or incinerators should be used for pigs, calves or other small animals.

What You Really Need To Know About Critical Animal Health Problems

THERE ARE two very important terms that are routinely used in developing a knowledge of animal diseases and health care of animals. They are "normal animal" and "disease."

A normal animal may be defined as one in which all body processes are working together in harmony and all body systems are working at their functional peak.

Any deviation from this normal condition then defines disease. The physical appearance, attitude and behavior of an animal indicates how it feels.

It isn't necessarily true that a normal, healthy looking animal is healthy. Therefore, a disease can be further defined as any deviation from normal with or without visible signs or symptoms.

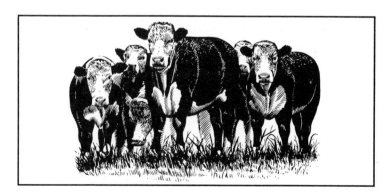

Disease Causes

Disease in livestock can be caused by several factors. Most livestock diseases are caused by one or a combination of two or more of the following:

Bacteria
Fungus
Heredity
Poisons
Virus
Injury
Nutrition
Parasites
Protozoa

Certain factors such as management, stress and weather are also said to be causes of diseases due to the fact that they weaken the animal's resistance to diseases. This weakening allows one or more of the specific disease-causing agents to produce a disease.

Disease Causing Agents

The following items highlight the various types of disease causing agents which are typically found in various kinds of farm animals.

Bacteria

Bacteria are one-cell plants which are microscopic in size. Bacteria are generally classified into three groups:

Harmless bacteria are frequently found in the air,

water, soil and also in the animal's body.

Beneficial bacteria are found in soil where they help maintain fertility, in the intestinal tract of all animals and in the rumen of cattle, where they help convert feeds into usable nutrients.

Harmful bacteria are those that cause disease, food spoilage and destroy other valuable products. The harmful bacteria that cause disease are called pathogenic bacteria.

Some bacteria have the ability to transform themselves into small, highly resistant spores. Spores are a resting stage that can often remain alive for years. Spores are highly resistant to heat and disinfectants. An example of a spore- caused disease is blackleg.

For bacteria to grow and multiply, they require moisture, suitable temperature, darkness and a food supply. Most pathogenic bacteria need living tissue to survive and multiply.

These conditions are simulated on an agar or culture plate. By placing a sample from a diseased animal on this media, a trained technician can identify the type of bacteria causing a disease. This test and a similar test called sensitivity testing can aid in the treatment of specific diseases.

Most bacterial diseases can be controlled by using antibiotics which are effective against a certain bacterial infection. Bacteria enter the body by various routes (respiration, eating, open wounds and in other ways) and cause disease by multiplying. Each species of pathogenic bacteria will attack a different area or tissue of the animal's body and produce varied symptoms.

As these bacteria grow and multiply, they produce toxins (poisons) that can interfere with the normal function or, in some cases, destroy the animal's body cells. The animal's body responds to bacterial infections by increasing the number of white blood cells in the circulating blood to fight the infection.

Examples of bacterial infections include:

Blackleg
Brucellosis
Dysentery
Mastitis
Vibriosis
E. coli
Erysipelas
Leptospirosis
Malignant Edema

Viruses

Viruses produce a disease process as a result of living and reproducing within a cell. As a consequence of the invading viruses, activity and production of toxins, they bring about the death of the host cell.

Viruses lack the ability to live and multiply anywhere but within a living host cell. After an animal has been exposed to pathogenic viruses, a variable period of time (several days to several weeks) elapses before the animal shows signs or symptoms of the disease. This interval of time is called the incubation period.

During the incubation period, the virus multiplies within the cell and gives rise to an alarming number of new, infective virus particles. As the virus multiplies, the infected cell's structure and function is destroyed. These cellular changes then give rise to the visible symptoms of the disease.

Viruses are minute microorganisms—so small they cannot be seen with an ordinary microscope. They enter the body in many ways, with the digestive tract and the respiratory system being the most significant. Another important route is through breaks in the skin or mucous membranes.

Infected mosquitoes feeding on a host is a fairly common avenue for transmitting sleeping sickness (equine enc eph alomyelitis) with horses. Rabies virus commonly enters through the bite wound inflicted by a rabid animal carrying the virus in its saliva. Viruses are responsible for causing a large proportion of all animal diseases.

Since viruses are not destroyed by antibiotics, the control of any virus is extremely difficult after the disease is established. Once viral diseases are established they virtually cannot be treated with present-day treatment products. Therefore, various methods must be employed to make the animal

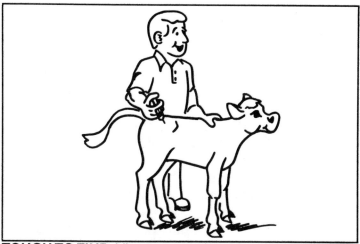

TOUGH TO FIND. Viruses enter the animal's body in many different ways. However, the digestive tract and the respiratory system are the two most common points for entry.

non-susceptible to any costly viral disease.

Such methods consist of colostrum feeding, vaccination and serum administration. These methods provide animal protection by either stimulating the production of antibodies or by simply providing protective antibodies.

Mechanical methods such as quarantine, sanitation or eradication serve to protect susceptible animals. Though not effective against the virus, using antibiotics will protect the animal against secondary bacterial infection that can result as the animal weakens to the virus disease.

Examples of viral diseases include:

    Bovine Virus Diarrhea (BVD)
    Hog Cholera
    Infectious Bovine Rhinotracheitis
    Parainfluenza3
    Pseudorabies
    Transmissible Gastroenteritis

Fungus

Thousands of fungi exist in nature and most are classified as either beneficial or harmless. Only a few are pathogenic in animals.

Feedstuffs contaminated with large quantities of fungi toxins (mycotoxins) fed to animals may lead to disease processes. These mycotoxins quite often may disturb the hormonal balance and sexual cycle of the animal or may even cause death.

Some types of fungi affect only surface tissue of the animal such as the skin and hair follicles. A common example of this type of infection is ringworm of man and animals. Treatment involves isolation of infected animals to prevent its spread and topical application with anti-fungal products.

Protozoa

These are the simplest of all animals. They are microscopic in size and usually represent only a single cell. While there are thousands of protozoa, only a few are pathogenic. Effective treatment products are available to rid an animal of most of the protozoa diseases, especially coccidia.

Examples of diseases caused by protozoa include:

Anaplasmosis
Coccidiosis (causing many deaths in poultry and
    gastrointestinal disturbances in cattle)
Trichmoniasis

Parasites

Parasites are a form of animal life which receive their nourishment at the expense of a large host animal. Parasites may take their nourishment by sucking blood (piercing or biting the skin) while

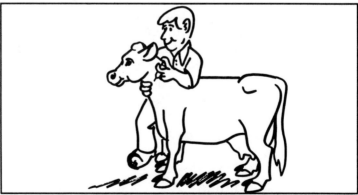

EXTERNAL PARASITES. This particular type of parasite gets its nourishment by sucking blood (by piercing or biting into the skin) or by burrowing deep into the animal's skin.

others burrow deep into the skin. These parasites are called external parasites. Parasites that derive their nutrition from within the animal's body, such as lungs, digestive tract, blood system, etc., are called internal parasites.

The size of these parasites may vary from microscopic to macroscopic (visible with naked eye) in size. Regardless of the size of the parasite, they can rob the animal of nutrients that could be used for milk or meat production.

In addition to causing lost production, other problems they cause are:

1 Act as vectors in spreading other diseases.

2 Weaken the animal, thus making it more susceptible to other diseases.

3 Cause tissue irritation and damage.

Losses from parasites can be effectively controlled by starting with a good sanitary environment and a regular treatment schedule. Treatment programs should be based upon the parasite to be treated, its stage of development and the selection of an effective product.

Examples of specific parasites are:

External Parasites...
Flies
Lice
Mange
Ticks

Internal Parasites...
Grubs
Lungworm
Nodular worm
Roundworm
Stomach worm
Tapeworm
Whipworm

Nutrition

This is the process of changing food into living tissue. To do this, the body needs many nutrients. Nutrients are substances in feed that are used to build and repair body tissue, provide a source of energy and regulate the body processes. When deficiencies of one or more nutrients exist for an extended period of time, it can cause the systems to function improperly.

Examples of nutritional diseases include:

Grass Tetany
Ketosis
Milk fever
Rickets

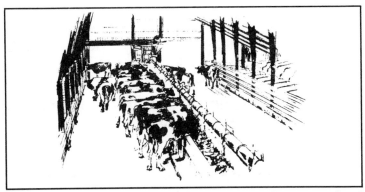

FEED RELATED DISEASES. If the ingredients you feed your animals are deficient in certain items, there are a number of nutritionally-related diseases which can result.

Poisons

These poisons can interfere with normal body processes, causing poor production or death. The two common sources of livestock poisoning result from consumption of poisonous plants or chemicals. Most poisons contain essential ingredients for body health, but become dangerous when taken in large quantities or over a long period of time.

Some chemical poisons are found in insecticides, herbicides, mineral mixtures and paint. The elements causing the poisoning are arsenic, lead, salt, organic phosphates, etc.

Examples of poisonous plants include:

Bracken fern
Poison hemlock
Oleander
White snake root

A Good Idea...

Many livestock producers tell us they utilize the easily-opened ring binding of this book to punch and insert clipped magazine articles, health remedy instruction sheets and their own personal animal health notes for handy barn or pasture reference in the future.

Chapter 3

The Transmission Of Infectious Diseases

THE AGENTS causing infectious diseases are transmitted in various ways. The nature of transmission is greatly dependent upon the characteristics of the microorganisms.

The three most common sources of disease-causing microorganisms are:

☛ Carrier animals.

☛ Contaminated feed and water.

☛ Soil borne.

While the sick animal is a prime source of disease-causing agents, animals that are convalescing (recovering from a disease) and occasionally even healthy animals which are fully recovered may still spread disease. Feedstuffs and water may be contaminated by carrier animals and they may serve as a source of disease agents.

Disease-causing microorganisms may lie dormant in the soil for years, yet become pathogenic in a susceptible animal. Examples of some of the diseases that lie dormant in the soil are erysipelas, tetanus and blackleg.

Escape Of The Microorganism From The Animal

Disease-causing microorganisms escape from the infected animal through routine body excretions. These microorganisms escape from the animal through moisture droplets in the exhausted air, nasal discharge, eye discharge, urine, feces, milking and other discharges such as cuts or scratches.

Since certain diseases tend to localize in certain systems of the animal's body, it is also known that they can escape by a routine excretion route. This becomes important in disease prevention, since some diseases can be relatively effectively controlled by routine cleaning and disinfection of the infective excretions.

Transfer Of The Microorganism To An Animal

Several methods exist which can transfer microorganisms to an animal. Quite often the microorganisms are transferred by one or more of the following:

- Direct contact (nose to nose)

- Droplet infection (airborne)

- Organisms on surfaces (food, water, equipment, boots, clothing, trucks)

- Feed, other livestock, rendering equipment and

trucks, buildings, pens, corrals, manure, etc.

• Stray dogs or cats, varmints, salespeople and vectors or carriers (mosquitoes, ticks, flies, etc.)

Once the microorganisms are transferred to an animal, the next step involves gaining entrance into the animal's system.

Entry Of Microorganisms Into Susceptible Animals

Microorganisms may enter an animal's body via a single route or a combination of routes. The animal may become infected by inhaling infective moisture droplets into its lungs, ingestion or swallowing of contaminated feedstuffs or water, become infected through a break in the skin, through the mucous membranes of the eye, nose, inside of the mouth or through reproductive organs.

Prevention And Control Of Infectious Diseases

Essentially, most control programs depend upon breaking the disease-spreading cycle by interfering with transmission at some stage. Control programs may include some or all of the following procedures:

Detection Of Infected Animal: To prevent the spread of disease-causing agents from an infected animal, it is first necessary to determine that animals are diseased. This can be done by a physical examination, the establishment of a diagnosis and/or serological testing.

Isolation: An animal identified to have an infectious disease should be separated from the remaining members of the herd or flock to avoid contact with susceptible animals.

New groups of animals should be penned separately for a minimum of 21 days. This 21-day period should be sufficient to allow a disease to break in the new group. (This period also allows animals to adjust slowly to the new environment).

Quarantine: This is an enforced isolation of an individual animal or herd in order to avoid all contact with unrestrained animals.

Treatment: Once a diagnosis of the causative disease agent is determined, treatment can be made. Several types of treatment products are available and they should be carefully selected for antiserums, antitoxins, antibiotics and chemotherapeutic agents—such as sulfas. Not only should these products be carefully selected, but they should also be used only as the label directions state.

Disposal Of Infected Animals: When animals are found dead, or when they are obviously near death, they should be posted by a veterinarian to determine the cause of death. The carcass should be disposed of by burying, cremating or having it picked up by a rendering truck.

Destruction Of Microorganisms In An External Environment

Follow these steps to make sure you have eliminated costly and dangerous organisms from your farming or ranching operation:

1 After removing your animals from various lots, pens or corrals, leave these areas vacant for a period of time.

2 Premises should be cleaned of manure and other organic matter. Next, the building and equipment should be scrubbed with a soap-disinfectant solution. Any piece of equipment or materials that cannot be properly cleaned should be immediately discarded regardless of the cost.

3 Disinfection of the premises. An agent which

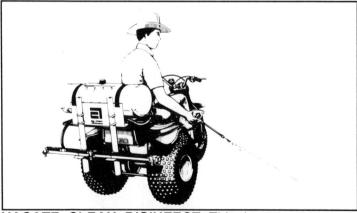

VACATE, CLEAN, DISINFECT. This three-step process is very essential if you are to eliminate most of the costly disease-causing organisms from your farming operation.

kills microorganisms is called a disinfectant, while the process of applying the disinfectant to microorganisms is called disinfection. Iodine based products are commonly used for disinfection and sanitation.

An ideal disinfection for areas which can be totally enclosed is the use of gaseous disinfectants. This process is called fumigation. The use of formaldehyde is commonly used as the disinfectant in fumigation.

Management And Sanitation

Sanitation is an important part of disease prevention and control. Sanitary practices vary from removing manure from the premises, disinfecting pens and stalls or veterinary equipment and the daily routines of such things as teat dipping.

However, the most important element in disease prevention and control is proper management. It is up to you to seek healthy livestock as additions to the herd, use only clean, disinfected trucks for transportation and isolate animals for observation upon arrival.

You should also oversee breeding, gestation and care of the newborn, as well as needing to oversee housing and nutrition.

It is also up to you to provide effective parasite control programs and programs of disease prevention by using vaccines and bacterins. In fact, programs of parasite control and disease prevention are what the this book's content will center around.

Chapter 4

Mechanisms Of Resistance To Disease

SEVERAL KEY TERMS are very important to any detailed understanding of the importance of knowing how disease resistance is developed in the animals which you raise. As a result, an understanding of these terms is essential for carrying out any highly successful animal health program.

Immunity

Immunity is the ability of an animal to resist disease. Certain animal species are completely non-susceptible to particular microorganisms that will cause disease in other species.

However, within a species, the immune state of an animal is a matter of degree. Furthermore, if resistance is not absolute, a large quantity of a virulent microorganism can usually overwhelm the resistance an animal possesses.

The immunity of an animal is another line of defense which a normal animal can use to fight infection. When bacteria and toxins cannot be destroyed by the lymphatic system and white blood cells, it is the immune system of the animal which fights the infection.

Antigen

An animal's body is under constant invasion by foreign protein substances called antigens. These antigens stimulate the body to build antibodies against disease.

Antibody

An antibody is a specific protein produced by the animal in response to the stimulation of an antigen. These specialized proteins are found in the blood and other body fluids that react with invading organisms or toxins to destroy them.

Classification Of Immunity

This all-important area can be further divided into several distinct types of immunity:

Natural Immunity

Each species of livestock has natural immunity or innate immunity to certain diseases. As an example, atrophic rhinitis affects only swine while blackleg affects only cattle. Many antibodies are not natural, but are formed in response to exposure to a disease agent.

Acquired Immunity

Acquired immunity is the immunity which a previously susceptible animal has developed or received. Acquired immunity can be broken down into two parts: passive immunity and active immunity.

Passive Immunity: This is so defined because the animal merely receives another animal's antibodies. Protection ceases once the supply is exhausted. Usually the immunity lasts for only a few weeks.

Two examples of passive immunization in an animal include feeding colostrum milk to a nervous animal or injecting serums produced by another animal. Passive immunity has an advantage over active immunity in cases of acute disease processes since it can provide the animal with immunity within minutes.

Active Immunity: As the name implies, active immunity requires some activity or action to produce an immunity. Active immunity is developed after an animal becomes diseased or from exposure through use of an immunizing agent.

The immune process in a susceptible animal usually takes 1 to 3 weeks after vaccination to build up significant numbers of antibodies in the circulating fluids. This is called the "primary immune response."

Over the following 4 to 6 weeks, the number of antibodies decreases. If an animal is exposed either by disease or revaccination to the same antigen the second time (whether a few weeks later or many years later), the immune response develops in 1 or 2 days and is far more lasting.

This is called the "second immune response." However, it is generally an immunity of long duration, possibly a year or even covering the entire life of an animal.

Vaccination

Vaccination is a valuable method of preventing disease. Vaccination with a veterinary biological product causes the development of antibodies against specific diseases or dangerous toxins without actually exposing the animal to the disease.

A long-lasting, active immunity is usually provided through vaccination. However, vaccination cannot give 100% animal protection because resistance to disease depends upon many factors. These include individual response to the vaccine, general health, nutritional status and the severity of a disease challenge or exposure. As a result, vaccination should not be considered the total answer for disease control. It should be supplemented with sanitary measures designed to prevent introduction and spread of infection.

Animals may be provided with passive immunity to a specific disease by means of antiserum. This form of immunity is short, usually lasting only 2 to 4 weeks. Protection is provided by the antibodies contained in the antiserum; when the supply of antibodies is exhausted or used up, protection ceases. Administration of an antiserum does not stimulate an animal's body to produce antibodies.

A pregnant animal that has developed active immunity to a disease may pass its antibodies to the newborn via colostrum and milk. This passive immunity lasts for only a short time after the animal is weaned.

Types Of Biological Products

Veterinary biological products are available in a wide variety of forms for specific uses and programs. The different types of products include:

Biologicals

Medicinal preparation made from living organisms and their products—serums, vaccines, antigens, antitoxins and bacterins.

Vaccines

In general, vaccines are used to provide relatively long immunity against disease. They are prepared from virulent, modified or dead viruses or bacteria.

Killed Virus Vaccine: This is produced by infecting an animal tissue with a specific virus. The virus is harvested at the height of the infection and is subjected to killing agents. When this vaccine is injected into an animal, the dead virus triggers production of antibodies.

Live Virus Vaccine: This is produced by growing a live culture of the virus from which a vaccine is prepared. The way it is injected into the animal is what gives this vaccine its immunizing quality and prevents it from actually causing the disease. For example, a vaccine quite often is placed on a scarification on the inside of the animal's thigh. It causes a small infection in this area that triggers antibody production throughout the animal.

Modified Live Virus Vaccine: This is an attenuated virus. Attenuation is a process of modifying a virus by growing it in another host. The virus then becomes less effective when given to the animal. When injected, it produces only a slight infection and stimulates production of antibodies.

Antiserum

This is produced by injecting a disease organism or its products into an animal. Dosages are gradually increased until large amounts are administered. The animal develops large numbers of antibodies in its own serums which are removed and prepared for injection into another animal. Protection antiserums generally last 2 or 3 weeks.

Antitoxin

This type of product is injected into an animal to neutralize toxins. Toxins are poisons produced by the growth activity of an invading bacteria such as a tetanus organism. Antitoxins produce short-lived immunity. They are produced by the body in much the same way as antibodies.

Toxoid

Such products contain neutralized toxins that stimulate an animal's body to produce antitoxins against a specific disease bacteria toxin. A common immunizing vaccine, tetanus, is a good example of this type of product.

Bacterin

This is a suspension of killed bacterial organisms used as an immunizing agent.

Chapter 5

Biologics For Animals

THE UNITED STATES has shown the world that control of animal diseases can certainly be a profitable venture. The animal health philosophy that prevails in this country is that if there is sufficient knowledge, technique and technicians, then diseases can be controlled and eradicated.

There is considerable evidence to support this view since cattle plague, glanders, foot and mouth, tick fever, vesicular exanthema and hog cholera have all been eradicated. Also close to eradication today are brucellosis and tuberculosis.

However, losses from many diseases and poor management practices continue to plague every livestock producer. The average livestock producer loses $2,500 to $3,500 a year due to disease. These losses are not just due to death of animals, but also result from poor feed efficiency, loss of gain and the cost of medicine and drugs.

In too many cases these losses are due to a combination of poor management practices and the failure to combine various facets of production into one sound livestock health management program.

Losses from disease in most cases are due to failure to adopt and employ recommended sound disease programs based on prevention. Too many livestock producers still handle disease problems after they occur—not before they occur.

One of the greatest livestock health abuses is seen in the care and use of biologics. Biologics are only one part of disease prevention. But because of lack of knowledge, carelessness and other practices, less than 50% of the vaccines used are effective.

For any livestock producer, a complete understanding of vaccines and vaccination procedures is necessary. There are over 230 kinds of vaccines, antiserums, antitoxins and other biologics on the market. They are all different and should be handled only as directed from the label.

Why Use Vaccines

Animals may inherit immunity to disease or they may acquire it. This power to resist development of disease can be acquired in two ways:

- As the result of successfully overcoming a natural infection.

- As a result of administering a biologic such as a vaccine.

Vaccination produces active and continuing immunity to a disease. No vaccine will provide 100% protection for all animals because animals differ in their response to vaccination and the amount of actual resistance they develop. However, proper vaccination usually provides an animal with enough protection to withstand exposure to a disease which would have been deadly without vaccination.

Many vaccines expose animals to mild attacks by specific disease organisms or the products of disease organisms contained in the biologic. This trig-

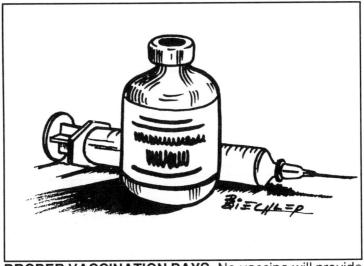

PROPER VACCINATION PAYS. No vaccine will provide 100% protection because animals differ in response to vaccination and amount of actual resistance they develop.

gers the animal's built-in system of defense against invading organisms. Antibodies—nature's disease fighters—are formed by the animal's body cells.

Then the battle begins. Even after overcoming the mild infection caused by the vaccine, the animal's body continues to produce antibodies. Within 1 or 2 weeks, enough antibodies are present to fight off future attacks by the same disease organism and active immunity is established.

Antiserums give passive immunity to disease organisms. This form of immunity is immediate but short-lived, usually lasting 2 to 4 weeks. Protection is provided by the antibodies contained in an antiserum.

Once the supply of antibodies is exhausted, protection for an animal ceases. The administration of an antiserum does not stimulate an animal's body to produce antibodies.

Types Of Vaccines

Vaccines are used to provide relatively long immunity against diseases. Vaccines are prepared from virulent, attenuated, weakened or dead viruses and bacteria.

A **killed-virus vaccine** is produced by injecting virus into a susceptible animal to cause the disease, killing the animal at the height of the infection and then preparing a vaccine from selected animal tissue. Formalin or other agents are used to inactivate the virus. An example of a killed-virus is Newcastle vaccine for poultry.

A **live-virus vaccine** is produced by inoculating a live virus into a medium, such as a chick embryo, permitting the virus to grow and then preparing the vaccine from infected fluids and tissues of the embryo.

A **modified live-virus vaccine** is prepared by processing the disease-causing virus in such a way that it no longer causes disease but stimulates immunity. An example would be Infectious Bovine Rhinotracheitis.

A **dessicated vaccine** is freeze-dried vaccine that must be reconstituted into a liquid state before use by addition of a diluent, usually distilled water. An example would be a live-virus rabies vaccine.

Monovalent vaccine and monovalent bacterin are biological products which stimulate immunity to two or more disease organisms. Examples include canine distemper-hepatitis vaccine and blackleg hemorrhagic septicemia bacterin.

Some vaccines are administered intranasally, others are given orally and most are administered parenterally (intramuscularly).

Antiserum

An antiserum can be used for quick protection against a disease. It contains large numbers of antibodies (disease fighters) that provide protection for 2 to 4 weeks. More lasting immunity is obtained against some diseases by using some vaccines simultaneously with antiserums. Large doses of an antiserum may also have a curative value. An example would be pseudorabies serum.

Antitoxin

An antitoxin is injected to neutralize poisons (toxins) caused by an invading disease organism and to produce short-lived immunity similar to that produced by an antiserum. Antitoxins contains large numbers of antibodies. Tetanus antitoxin would be a good example.

Bacterin

A bacterin is used to stimulate immunity against bacterial diseases. It contains a standardized number of killed bacteria. Upon injection, a bacterin causes an animal to produce antibodies which will fight future invasions of the same type of bacteria.

A mixed bacterin contains standardized numbers of four or more bacterial organisms. They are used to prevent conditions attributed to the organisms used in making the product. Examples are erysipelas bacterin or clostridial bacterins.

Diagnostic Agents

Diagnostics and diagnostic antigens are biologics used to detect and diagnose disease, either by causing a typical reaction following injection into an animal (diagnostic) or producing standard results in laboratory blood tests (diagnostic antigen). Examples include tuberculin antigen, mycoplasma gallisepticum antigen and pullorum antigen.

Administer Biologics Skillfully

Vaccinate only healthy animals. Chronic infections or the presence of parasites lowers an animal's resistance and could cause the vaccinated animal to have to fight off several diseases at the same time. Immunization will be adversely affected by anything that weakens the animal. This includes overwork, exposure to cold, lack of proper feed and shipment over long distances—especially during stormy weather.

To increase your chances for successful vaccination, eliminate as many adverse conditions as you can. Free animals of parasites, clear up chronic infections, eliminate deficiencies in the diet and protect them from cold and dampness.

Age also is an important factor in vaccination. Neither very young or very old animals respond as well to vaccination as those found between the two extremes. This is very important and is one aspect of management that is frequently ignored. In a recent survey, more than 50% of all calves were vaccinated for blackleg at too early of an age.

Follow-Up Is Very Important

Keep detailed records of vaccination, including serial numbers of products. This information could later be very important in tracing the cause of any unsatisfactory results.

Never save opened, unused portions of biologics. These can easily lose potency and become impure and unsafe.

Safely dispose of empty biologic containers and unused portions by burning them or burying them at least 18 in. deep on level land. Watch your animals closely for 2 or 3 weeks after vaccination.

Reactions such as swelling or lesions often occur after administration of some vaccines, such as anthrax or brucella vaccines. If reactions persist or if your animals show general symptoms of disease, call your veterinarian.

If you do the vaccinating yourself, there are several important rules to follow:

☛ Store biologics in subdued light. Keep them refrigerated at all times, even in the field. Never let them freeze.

☛ Use only sterilized vaccinating equipment. Dirty needles, etc., have caused a great deal of trouble and skin abscesses.

☛ Carefully cleanse and disinfect the inoculation site before vaccinating.

☛ Be sure you know the site of administration. If directions state "intramuscular," have your veterinarian supply you with the right length and size of needle. Where vaccines are deposited can have a big impact on the degree of protection obtained.

☛ Never mix biologics and never use outdated vaccines.

☛ Dispose of empty biologic containers and unused portions by burning immediately after use.

Do It Right

Vaccination of animals is a very important part of any disease prevention program. It has, however, been grossly abused and misunderstood, thus lessening the effectiveness of vaccine.

For the welfare of the animal and pet industry, it is hoped that correct vaccination procedures are followed. In case of doubt, call one who knows—your veterinarian.

Approximate Measures

1/2 ounce (fluid)	4 teaspoons
1/2 ounce (fluid)	1 tablespoonful
4 ounces (fluid)	1 teacupful
8 ounces (fluid)	1 glassful
1 c.c.	16 drops
4 c.c.	1 teaspoonful

Chapter 6

Animal Health Supplies You Need On Hand

THERE ARE A number of animal health supplies you should have on hand for emergencies and the treatment of minor ailments. However, remember that many of these products are perishable and become out of date while others have a long shelf life.

Some products are poisonous and thus should not be kept where they can become part of the animal's feed supply or be handled by children. A separate cupboard or chest should be provided for the storage of these supplies and it should be kept padlocked.

Never use any product that does not have an attached label or directions. Never use a product that is outdated. All biologics should be kept refrigerated. Your veterinarian is the logical person to aid you in stocking your critical animal health supply inventory.

Basic Animal Health Needs

The following equipment is recommended for each particular species of livestock:

Cattle

Nose lead with rope
Lariot
Trocar and cannula
Obstetrical chains
Castrating knife
Udder ointment
Wound dressing
Mastitis treatment
Dry cow treatment
Emascultome
Syringes and needles
Disinfectants
Alcohol—isopropyl
Vaseline
Tincture of iodine
Mineral oil
Bandages and tape
Thermometer
Spray cans of insecticides
Dehorning device or paste

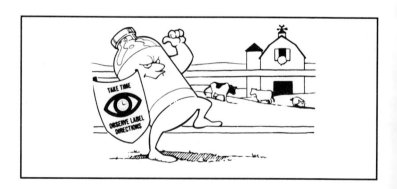

Swine

Hog catcher
Pig teeth nippers
Syringes and needles
Castrating knife
Ear notcher and hog ringer

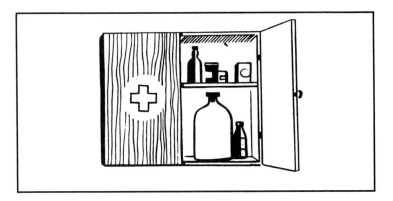

Sheep

Drenching equipment
Syringes
Docking tool
Foot knives
Marking crayons

Horse

Halters
Ropes
Wound treatments

Refrigerated Storage Is Needed

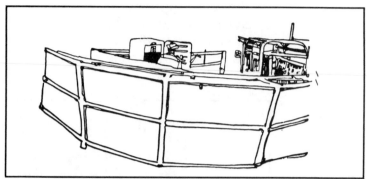

KEEP THEM COOL. Biological products should be stored in a refrigerator. Otherwise, they will lose their strength and won't be able to do the job with your animals when needed.

All biologics should be prescribed by the veterinarian and stored in a refrigerator. Antibiotics, sulfonamides, pinkeye treatments, powders and insecticides should be obtained from your veterinarian and be labeled properly with withholding times clearly visible. Availability of treatments and biologics is such that an inventory is not necessary because of the specificity of treatment and out-dating that can occur.

Prescription drugs are those used by or under the supervision of your veterinarian. These drugs can be obtained only from a licensed veterinarian. Caution should be used if prescription drugs are found to be available from other sources.

Insecticides are recommended for various species. However, remember that using just one insecticide will not serve for all species of animals. Certain insecticides frequently are no longer approved. Purchase insecticides as needed. Always adhere to labelled withdrawal times.

Chapter 7

First Aid Tips For Treating Your Animals

ANIMAL OWNERS can certainly do a great deal of administering to their animals in case of suspected illness or injury. But in all cases, animal owners should know a veterinarian, his telephone number and his office location.

Most veterinarians welcome the delivery of animals to their clinic if at all possible. This is particularly true when only one animal is ailing. Further, a veterinarian who knows you, your animals and your method of management can render the best possible service.

In most cases, the degree of management that prevails usually dictates the level of health in animals. The owner who knows and accepts the responsibility of animal ownership or custody and provides proper nutrition, environment and care will have little, if any, illness and injury to his or her animals. The greatest abuse of animal welfare is the animal that is allowed to become parasitized, sick and is not attended to when needed. Letting a sick animal go too long is a common complaint that veterinarians have about animal owners.

There are a number of chapters in this book that show how you can identify sick animals and properly render first aid. However, this information in no way is given to imply that veterinary service is not needed.

Recording Body Temperature

The temperature of an animal will give you an indication of the state of health of the animal. The following are the most important steps in recording the temperatures of animals:

☞ The temperature of all animals are taken rectally, therefore, the animals must be restrained.

☞ Shake the mercury column down until the reading is at 95 to 97 degrees.

☞ Dip the bulb of the thermometer in vaseline or a lubricating jelly.

☞ Insert the thermometer into the rectum. If necessary, clean out large deposits of feces so the bulb of the thermometer lies next to the lining of the rectum.

☞ Leave in for 3 minutes. Either tie the thermometer to the tail of the animal or hold it in place while recording the temperature.

☞ Animals will have a higher temperature on hot days or after they have become excited. Account for this variation and repeat the temperature reading if necessary.

☞ Use the following chart to determine whether the thermometer reading you have obtained is normal.

☞ Clean off the thermometer with soap and water

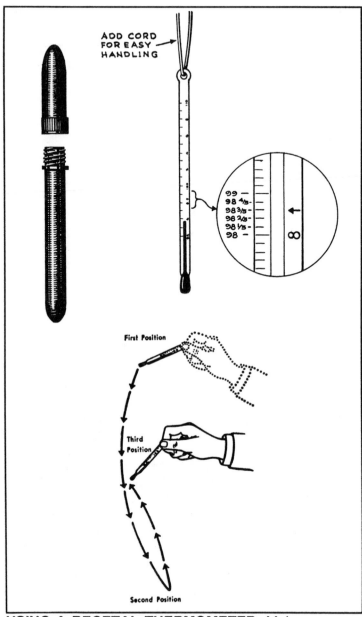

ADD CORD
FOR EASY
HANDLING

First Position

Third
Position

Second Position

USING A RECETAL THERMOMETER. Make sure you always keep thermometers in the cases they come with for needed protection. Running a string or cord through the loop on the end of the thermometer makes it easier to use. Bottom diagrahm shows the proper procedure for shaking your thermometer to get it back to the normal temperature.

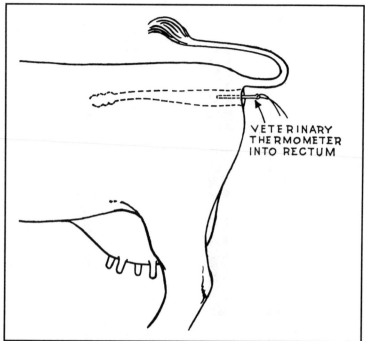

VETERINARY
THERMOMETER
INTO RECTUM

INSERTING THE THERMOMETER. The thermometer should be inserted bulb first into the rectum. There is no danger of breaking if normal care is taken, but be sure the thermometer bulb is touching the rectal wall or fecal material so gas pockets can not form. If the bulb is in a gas pocket, the thermometer will often give a reading which is below the actual temperature.

Let the thermometer find its own direction. If you hold it stifly, it may poke inside and cause the animal pain. The thermometer bulb should be inserted deep into the rectum, at least 2 or 3 inches but still leaving enough hanging out for its recovery. The bulb is the only part of the thermometer which registers the temperature. There generally is less chance for breakage if the thermometer is inserted well into the rectum rather than when it is only partly inserted.

and store in a convenient place.

☛ Do not wash the thermometer in hot water.

Rectal Temperatures

The following are animal temperatures to use in evaluating the health of your animals:

Dairy Cattle

Average temperature—101.6.
Normal range of temperature—100.4 to 102.8.
Temperatures which indicate illness under normal conditions—103.0 and rising.
Temperatures which indicate illness under conditions of hot weather, excitement and/or extensive exercise—104.0 and rising.

Beef Cattle

Average temperature—101.0.
Normal range of temperature—98.0 to 102.4.
Temperatures which indicate illness under normal conditions—103.4 and rising.
Temperatures which indicate illness under conditions of hot weather, excitement and/or extensive exercise—104.4 and rising.

Hogs

Average temperature—102.4.
Normal range of temperature—101.6 to 103.6.
Temperatures which indicate illness under normal conditions—104.4 and rising.
Temperatures which indicate illness under conditions of hot weather, excitement and/or extensive exercise—105.4 and rising.

Horses

Average temperature—99.8.
Normal range of temperature—99.0 to 100.8.
Temperatures which indicate illness under normal conditions—101.4 and rising.
Temperatures which indicate illness under conditions of hot weather, excitement and/or extensive exercise—102.0 and rising.

Sheep

Average temperature—102.2.
Normal range of temperature—100.8 to 103.8.
Temperatures which indicate illness under normal conditions—104.4 and rising.
Temperatures which indicate illness under conditions of hot weather, excitement and/or extensive exercise—105.4 and rising.

Goats

Average temperature—102.0.
Normal range of temperature—100.6 to 102.0.
Temperatures which indicate illness under normal conditions—103.0 and rising.
Temperatures which indicate illness under conditions of hot weather, excitement and/or extensive exercise—104.0 and rising.

Dogs

Average temperature—101.4.
Normal range of temperature—100.4 to 102.4.
Temperatures which indicate illness under normal conditions—103.0 and rising.
Temperatures that indicate illness in hot weather or hard exercise—104.0 and rising.

Chapter 8

Making Proper Use Of Disinfectants

DISINFECTION IS very important in controlling the accumulation and spread of disease-causing microorganisms. This is especially true in modern livestock and poultry confinement buildings where continuous use and high concentrations of animals may result in a condition referred to as "disease buildup."

As disease-producing bacteria, fungi and parasite eggs accumulate in the environment, disease problems can be transmitted to each successive group of animals which is raised. Dairy calf-raising facilities, swine buildings and poultry houses are especially vulnerable. Thorough cleaning and disinfection often provide the only successful solution to breaking the disease cycle and controlling the problem.

Principles Of Disinfection

Because organic matter in dirt and manure inactivates certain disinfectants and protects infective microorganisms from germicidal activity, good cleaning is certainly necessary for proper disinfection.

Simple scrubbing or a high velocity stream of water can do an excellent cleaning job, but use of detergent solutions will hasten dirt and manure removal, increase the wetting speed and break down organic matter into small particles which will easily wash away.

While portable steam generators or "steam jennies" are useful for cleaning dirty surfaces, they do not kill organisms effectively. However, the removal of accumulated grime permits disinfectants to more easily penetrate and kill infective organisms.

Various commercially available chemical disinfectants have many different mechanisms of action as well as different spectra of activity. Many factors must be weighed in choosing a proper disinfectant for a particular job.

For example, a germicide intended for disinfecting a building should work well in the presence of organic matter, be compatible with soaps and detergents, be harmless to building materials and be relatively nontoxic. For disinfection of dairy barns, however, a germicide must have the additional quality of being free of strong odor to minimize the possibility of tainting milk. A disinfectant suitable for decontaminating a building might also be too toxic for use in sanitizing food and water utensils.

Disinfectants Compared

The following is intended as a guide to the selection of currently used disinfectants.

Alkalies

These have been used as germicidal agents since antiquity. A pH greater than 9 will inhibit most bacteria and destroy many viruses.

- Lye (soda lye) contains approximately 94% sodium hydroxide, a very effective disinfectant. For disinfectant purposes, lye should be applied as a 2% solution in hot or boiling water (1 lb. of lye to 5.5 gal. of water). To destroy resistant spores of the anthrax organism, a 5% solution is recommended.

- Concentrated lye is a caustic poison and must be handled with care. Solutions of lye can injure painted or varnished surfaces and textiles if allowed to remain in contact for very long. Lye does not injure bare wood, enamelware, earthenware or any of the common metals except aluminum.

- Lime (calcium oxide, quicklime) is one of the least expensive disinfectants and is reasonably good for use around livestock. Powdered lime may be scattered about yards or lots or swept over concrete floors for general disinfection. Since it tends to dry the skin and hooves of animals and sometimes causes cracks which invite foot rot, excessive amounts of lime on concrete floors should be avoided.

Surfactants

These surface-active agents are chemical compounds which lower the surface tension of aqueous solutions and thus promote wetting.

- Soaps, in general, are mild disinfectants. They are antibacterial against certain gram-positive organisms such as the common skin-inhibiting species, but are much less effective against gram-negative microorganisms associated with fecal contamination. The primary value of soaps as disinfectants is in facilitating the mechanical removal of contaminated organic matter.

- Quaternary ammonium compounds are surfactants commonly used as general antibacterial disinfectants with dairy, meat-packing and food-handling equipment. They do not possess substantial viricidal, fungicidal or sporicidal action and are used chiefly as sanitizing rinses for eating, drinking and dairy utensils after mechanical cleaning. These compounds are not suitable for disinfection of buildings since they are readily inactivated by organic matter. Since they are also neutralized by soaps, surfaces to be disinfected with them should be thoroughly rinsed.

Halogens

A number or halogens, such as chlorine, iodine and halogen compounds, have potent antibacterial effects. In the presence of organic matter, iodine is more active than chlorine.

- The activity of iodine solutions is directly related to the amount of free iodine present. Tincture of iodine is a 2% solution of elementary iodine in alcohol and is a very effective antiseptic. Strong tincture of iodine (7%) has a greater antibacterial action but is more irritating to tissue.

- Iodophors are combinations of iodine and solubilizing compounds, usually nonionic detergents. They are non-staining, non-irritating and are largely free from the risk of producing hypersensitivity. Iodophors, sometimes referred to as "tamed iodines," are commonly used to disinfect dairy utensils and equipment and for teat dipping after milking. Iodophors prepared for use on equipment contain phosphoric acid and should not be used on skin.

- Chlorine has a rapid action against bacteria, spores, fungi and viruses. Its activity, however, is substantially reduced by the presence of organic matter so preliminary cleaning is always essential before chlorine disinfection is undertaken.

- Solutions of sodium hypochlorite, similar to those used as laundry bleaches, are commonly used to disinfect dairy utensils. Such solutions decompose upon exposure to light and should be kept protected.

- A 2% solution of calcium hypochlorite (bleaching powder or chloride of lime) is a cheap but effective disinfectant for buildings and utensils. Its action, however, is readily dissipated by organic matter and careful cleaning should precede its use.

- Powdered chlorinated lime may be dusted directly on contaminated livestock quarters to serve as a powerful deodorant as well as a good disinfectant. It should be stored in airtight con-

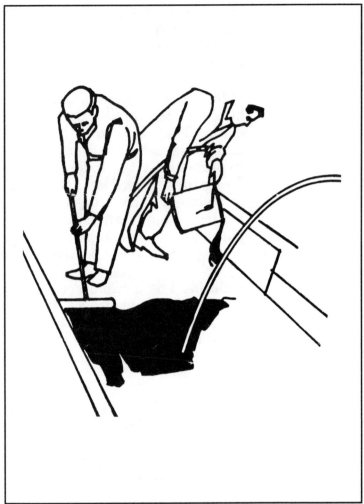

NO EASY CHOICES. Many different disinfectant products are available—each with distinct advantages and disadvantages. Selecting the right disinfectant for a particular cleaning job is very important to you and it will involve the special consideration of a rather large number of factors.

tainers because it deteriorates upon exposure to air. Chloramines are organic chlorine compounds which release chlorine slowly and exert a prolonged bactericidal effect. They are less toxic and irritating than the hypochlorites.

Coal And Wood Tar Derivatives

There are several types of these products that are very useful in disinfecting animal buildings and facilities:

- Phenol (carbolic acid) is reasonably effective in destroying most common types of bacteria, but is too expensive and toxic for general use. Concentrations in excess of 2% phenol are dangerous for all species of animals, particularly cats, because of absorption through the skin.

- Cresol is relatively inexpensive and efficient as a disinfectant. It is not readily soluble in water and hot water should be used for preparing solutions.

- Saponated cresol preparations, such as "Lysol," are mixtures of cresol with soap which form more readily soluble solutions for easier application. Cresylic compounds, in general, are not suitable for use in dairy barns because their strong and persistent odor may contaminate milk. The U.S. Agricultural Research Service suggests the use of an acceptable cresol or saponated cresol compound for disinfecting animal quarters, carriers and premises. A dilution of 4 oz. per gal. of water is recommended. Pressure spraying is the easiest, most efficient method of application.

- Sodium orthophenylphenate is a coal tar derivative which has been recognized as an official disinfectant by the U.S. Department of Agriculture, primarily because of its effectiveness against tuberculosis organisms. It is readily soluble in water, has potent germicidal activity and is active in the presence of detergents and moderate amounts of organic material. Because it irritates the eyes and mucous membranes, simple precautions must be observed during its use. Since it has no objectionable odor, it is suitable for use in dairy barns.

Miscellaneous Disinfectants

You also have a wide choice of different products in this category to choose from for disinfecting facilities:

- Hydrogen peroxide solutions release free oxygen rapidly upon contact with mucous membranes or denuded surfaces which provide the enzyme catalase. When hydrogen peroxide is applied to a wound containing exudate, its effervescence in the recesses of the wound is beneficial in the mechanical removal of pus and organic debris. In infected tissue, hydrogen peroxide is probably of more value as a cleansing agent than as a germicide.

- Common alcohols are good solvents, antiseptics and disinfectants. Ethyl alcohol (ethanol, grain alcohol) is commonly used as a dilution of 70% by weight or 78% by volume for cleaning and disinfecting skin, syringes, instruments, etc. This concentration has greater germicidal activity than either more concentrated or more dilute solutions.

- Isopropyl alcohol has antibacterial properties similar to ethyl alcohol and is generally used in the same concentration. Isopropyl alcohol, being nonintoxicating, is exempt from the special tax which must be paid on ethyl alcohol. For disinfecting purposes, it is cheaper and just as effective.

- Chlorhexidine ("Nolvasan") is a synthetic compound which has proven useful in disinfecting contaminated equipment and premises, sanitizing udder cloths and milking equipment, as a topical germicide for wound treatment and in teat dipping. It is active against a variety of microorganisms, is not appreciably inactivated by small quantities of organic matter and is relatively nontoxic. Chlorhexidine is commercially available as a 2% solution as well as in other forms.

- Formaldehyde solution can be purchased as an aqueous solution containing about 40% formaldehyde gas, commonly known by the name "Formalin." A concentration of 4% formaldehyde gas is an excellent, reliable disinfectant and is lethal to anthrax spores within 15 minutes.

- Fumigation with formaldehyde has been popular in large poultry houses and swine units. Proper disinfection depends on a long period of exposure at proper concentration and humidity. Because the gas tends to condense at low temperatures, fumigation with formaldehyde is unreliable below 65 degrees Fahrenheit. Buildings should be thoroughly cleaned before fumigation and must be aired for 12 to 24 hours before reuse.

There are actually two basic methods of fumigating facilities with formaldehyde gas:

☛ The first employs using wide bottom buckets placed approximately every 10 ft. through the length of the building. In each receptacle, 175 grams (10 level tablespoons) of potassium permanganate is placed, then 12 oz. (1 1/2 cups) of a 40% solution of formaldehyde (formalin) is poured over it. Under proper conditions this mixture will generate enough formaldehyde gas to disinfect 1,000 cu. ft. of space.

☛ The second method employs a white powder, paraformaldehyde, and commercially available electric heating units which release the gas from the powder. With either method, the floor should be moistened about 15 minutes before fumigation and the building must be kept tightly closed for at least 8 hours.

No Easy Choice

There are a number of readily-available disinfectants, each having various advantages and disadvantages. The proper choice of a disinfectant for a particular job is a very important decision and involves consideration of many factors.

Thorough cleaning, including the use of detergents, is an essential step which must precede the proper application of germicidal agents. Frequent manure removal, routine cleanliness and proper disinfection are management procedures which can provide great dividends in healthy, productive livestock. These simple measures will reduce the hazards of disease buildup that significantly increase death losses, reduce growth rates or feeding efficiency and decrease your profits.

Chapter 9

Water Quality For Your Animals Is Very Critical

APPROXIMATELY 60% to 85% of the daily nutrition of farm livestock is represented by consumption of a valuable, low-cost ingredient—water. The fat-free adult body water content is relatively constant for many species of animals, averaging 71% to 73% of the total body weight.

The total water supply used by an animal comes from five principal sources:

☛ Drinking water.

☛ Water contained in or on feed.

☛ Metabolic water produced by oxidation of organic nutrients.

☛ Water liberated from polymerization reactions such as condensation of amino acids to peptides.

☛ Preformed water associated with the tissues which are catabolized during a period of negative energy balance.

Obviously, our concerns for water quality must be concentrated on the first source, drinking water.

Animals Need Lots Of Water

The amount of water consumed by an individual animal actually depends on several variables:

- Type of ration.

- Amount of feed intake.

- Temperature.

- Humidity.

- Physical form of feed.

- Species of animal.

- Production state of animal.

- Size of animal.

- Water quality.

The accompanying table illustrates water consumption rates for various species of animals under "normal" conditions. The figure shown for dairy cattle will, of course, vary dramatically with milk production. Estimates range from 4 to 6 lbs. of water needed for each 1 lb. of milk that is produced. Thus, the cow that produces 100 lbs. of milk per day could easily consume 50 gal. of water daily.

Since water quality directly affects water consumption and since the first effect of water restriction, whether voluntary or involuntary, is to reduce the feed consumption and thus efficiency, the importance of an adequate on-farm supply of high quality

Amount Of Water Which "Normal" Animals Drink

Animal Species	Weight Of Animal	Water Consumed Per Day
Cattle	350 lbs.	1-5 gal.
	750 lbs.	10-15 gal.
	1,000 lbs.	20 gal.
Sheep	20 lbs.	1/2 gal.
	40-60 lbs.	1/3 gal.
	100-200 lbs.	1/4 gal.
Swine	20-40 lbs.	1/4-1/2 gal.
	100 lbs.	3/4-1 gal.
	200 lbs.	1 1/4-1 3/4 gal.
Dairy cow		15-25 gal.
Chickens	100 head	3-3 1/2 gal.
Turkeys	100 head	17 gal.

water becomes extremely critical.

Low quality water may cause problems in two ways. Palatability may be lower, thus water consumption will decrease.

Or toxic substances may be present. Some toxic substances do not reduce palatability and are thus potentially even more harmful than those reducing palatability. Substances that may prove toxic in drinking water include fluorine, molybdenum, nitrates, selenium and other specific trace substances of heavy concentrations. Bacterial contamination of the water supply can also increase its toxic properties.

In addition to toxic substances, water may contain other compounds that render it unpalatable. An example is alkali water containing high concentrations of potassium, sodium and calcium carbonates. Waters high in saline are less palatable than nonmineral water. Saline salts are sodium, calcium, magnesium and potassium in the bicarbonate, chloride or sulfate forms.

The palatability of water is greatly enhanced by the presence of carbon dioxide as shown by the wide popularity of bottled carbonated drinks. When opened, they quickly become less palatable due to the escape of the gas. Rainwater, distilled water and boiled water have a "flat" taste due to their low carbon dioxide content. Freshly drawn deep well water loses some of its carbon dioxide on standing and becomes less palatable.

Water Contaminants

A partial listing of some water contaminants, their effects on animals and what can be done about them by livestock producers follows:

Total Dissolved Solids—Hardness

Most domestic farm animals can tolerate a total dissolved solid concentration in the range of 15,000 to 17,000 mg per liter. Salts in amounts of 5,000 parts per million (ppm) affect palatability for animals, and if consumed, will often produce considerable weight loss and costly diarrhea.

Probably more important than the levels of dissolved solids is the actual chemical composition of the solids. These sources of hardness will be discussed separately. However, it is not always desirable that water be completely free from minerals that make it hard. Soft water is likely to be corrosive, especially if the pH value is very low.

Water softening is the usual means of removing hardness from water. However, certain precautions are needed here, as the mode of action of a water softener is to displace the dissolved solids with sodium from salt. If the level of dissolved solids (hardness) is significant, more harm may be done by introducing water with an extremely high concentration of sodium, which could result from the softening of very hard water. The sodium/potassium/magnesium relationships are just now becoming known and it appears that definite ratios must exist between these metals for maximum production regardless of the source.

A newer, more sophisticated method of removing hardness from water is reverse osmosis. Osmosis is the natural passage of a liquid through a semipermeable membrane during which the liquid flows from a state of low concentration of solids or impurities to a state of relatively high concentration.

To purify a liquid by the osmotic process, it must be reversed to make the liquid flow from a state of high concentration of solids to a low concentration. This is done by applying pressure to the high concentration side of the membrane and the result is a purified liquid. This process is capable of rejection of 90% to 95% of the total solids in the water including particulate matter, colloidal suspensions, organic matter, pyrogens and bacteria. This type of purification system may be the one of choice when water is harder than 250 ppm.

Nitrates

The entire nitrate problem, its effects on production and reproduction, safe limits, complications with other nitrogen sources and desirable methods of removal and/or neutralization are all subjects of considerable controversy at the present time.

Nitrates, if ingested in large enough quantities, can be absorbed as nitrites. In this form in the blood, they will reduce hemoglobin to methemoglobin, thus reducing the oxygen- carrying capacity of the blood.

In ruminant animals, a nitrate problem may appear as a vitamin A deficiency. Supplementing the ration with additional amounts of vitamin A and phosphorus will restore the nutritional balance, as it will for all species.

The range of arbitrarily unsafe nitrate in the water probably lies between 50 and 100 ppm. The apparent interference with normal nutrition, gestation, growth and health begins at about 100 ppm nitrates. The U.S. Public Health Service sets 45 ppm of nitrate as the upper limit for a safe water supply.

There are many sources of nitrates in water and there are probably many more unidentified sources. Increased crop fertilization can contribute to nitrate contamination of the water. Surface contamination from manure and barnyards as runoff is probably the most common, troublesome source for poorly located shallow wells or ponds. Nitrates may build up in deep water supplies by being leached down through the soils.

Little is known of the variation in nitrate concentration in a well. Test reports indicate that nitrate levels may fluctuate widely. Nitrate levels are generally the highest following wet periods and lowest, even down through zero, during dry periods of the year. Testing during only dry periods may cause a false sense of security.

When nitrates are found in the water supplies, their removal may be difficult and expensive. Since they are dissolved, they cannot be filtered out through the use of ordinary filters. A relatively new, commercially available unit removes nitrate ions from water by means of strongly basic anion exchangers. This unit also has the capability of removing sulfates from water.

If nitrates and/or nitrites are discovered in a water source, certain compensating changes can be made to the nutrition of the affected animals to help neutralize the effects of these substances. These changes could include:

Increasing vitamin A levels, since nitrates apparently interfere with normal vitamin A metabolism and storage.

Increasing the caloric density of the ration (more grain), since nitrates from feed are usually found in the stem of the plant and because the reduction of nitrates to ammonia requires energy which would then reduce the available energy for production and reproduction.

Biological Properties

These water-borne pathogenic microorganisms may be divided into five different groups:

- Enteric vegetative bacteria, such as Salmonella and Shigella.

- Viruses, such as hepatitis, polio and coxsackie.

- Spore-forming bacteria, such as Bacillus Anthracis.

- Intestinal Protozoa, such as Endamoeba Histolytica.

- Worms such as the cercariae of the schistosomemes.

For over 50 years, the accepted criterion of the sanitary quality of water has been the absence or presence of the coliform group of bacteria. This index is a criterion only for intestinal bacteria and does not apply to the presence of other enteric pathogens.

These viruses are more resistant to disinfection with chlorine than are coliforms. The standard chlorine doses that are recommended and used by municipalities in public water supplies cannot inactivate viruses without excessively long contact periods which are not usually available in municipal systems.

Although all coliform bacteria are not pathogens, many do possess this potential. Their presence indicates infectious bacteria and viruses may also be present. Most diseases can be transmitted from contaminated water to animals.

Criteria Used For Determining The Quality Of Drinking Water For Livestock And Poultry
(Inorganic elements and compounds)

Aluminum	5 mg/L
Arsenic	.2 mg/L
Beryllium	No limit
Boron	5 mcg/L
Cadmium	50 mg/L
Chromium	1 mg/L
Copper	.5 mg/L
Fluorine	2 mg/L
Iron	No limit
Lead	.1 mg/L
Manganese	No limit
Mercury	1 mcg/L
Molybdenum	No limit
Nitrates and nitrites	100 ppm
Nitrites	10 ppm
Selenium	.05 mg/L
Vanadium	.1 mg/L
Zinc	25 mg/L

The only sure way of identifying microorganisms in the water is by actual incubation of a water sample on an appropriate medium. The presence of bacteria can be predicted through observation of other qualitative tests made on the water sample.

Bacteria accompanies nutrients found in water suppliles such as nitrites, nitrates and phosphates, proportionally. If these nutrient levels are high, the bacteria level will also be high. However, waters containing nitrates may show no evidence of bacterial pollution by either animal or human waste.

By far the most popular method of destroying bacteria in a water supply is through chlorination. This can be accomplished in several ways:

Low levels of chlorine can be used if the water is exposed to the chlorine for a period of time prior to consumption. This time period varies according to the degree of contamination, pH of water and the temperature of water.

Higher levels of chlorine may be used and thus exposure time can be greatly reduced. This method is referred to as "superchlorination" and will be discussed in detail later. Boiling water, although not practical on a large scale, will disinfect the water.

Other additives or treatments for contaminated water which have proven successful include iodine, ozone, exposure to ultraviolet rays and exposure to ultrasonics. Filters may also be used, but they should not be substitutes for disinfecting the water. After bacteria have been destroyed, objectionable chlorine taste and odor can be removed by an activated carbon filter.

pH Content

Acid water corrodes pumps, pipe, tanks and fixtures. This dissolving action damages iron pipes and leaves a reddish or bluish discoloration on sinks, tubs, etc. Correcting the acid content of your water can add years to the life of your plumbing system. Acid water is neutralized by feeding a neutralizing agent into the water.

The two most common neutralizing agents are soda

ash or caustic soda. Neither of these add hardness to the water as do neutralizing filters. Acid may also be removed by aeration. The water should be broken into small droplets so the maximum surface is presented to the air.

Alkalinity is found in most water supplies and comes from bicarbonates, carbonates and hydroxides which give a soda taste to the water. It usually promotes the growth of bacteria and may cause precipitation of scale in water pipes and heaters. Alkalinity can be created by chlorination, demineralization, distillation and precipitation.

Chlorides

Alone, chlorides are not harmful unless found in large quantities (over 200 ppm). Chlorides unite with sodium forming brine wells and other salts which render some well water useless. The salts can be removed, but the removal of chlorides requires an expensive process of distillation and/or demineralization. Levels of 50 to 100 ppm are more palatable to livestock.

Human supplies are usually classed as objectionable when more than 5 ppm of chlorine are present. Precoat carbon filters can be used to protect water for human consumption from amoebic cysts and to dechlorinate the water.

Although some work indicates that chlorine, in highly concentrated doses, is toxic and injurious to the mucous membrane of the throat, actual cases of ingestion of large amounts of chlorine prove that individuals have a relatively high degree of tolerance to highly chlorinated water.

Sulfates

Excessive sulfates (over 500 ppm) in water can cause scours in baby pigs, beef calves and dairy calves. Sulfates over 1,000 ppm may have a cathartic effect on livestock, particularly younger animals. However, all animals appear to be able to develop a tolerance to constant level of sulfates (2,000 ppm to 2,500 ppm) after a period of time.

Since sodium sulfates and magnesium sulfate are well known laxatives, the effects of water sulfates in these forms are usually quite noticeable. Until recently, demineralization, distillation and precipitation were the only methods of removal with precipitation being the most economical. However, there are now commercial units available that effectively and economically remove sulfates from water.

Phosphates

When phosphates are found in rural well waters in large amounts, this usually means pollution. Phosphates by themselves are harmless.

However, they are a source of nutrition for bacteria and their presence should alert one to the probability of bacterial contamination. Chlorination is the treatment of choice.

Iron

As little as .3 ppm in water supplies will cause the familiar brown staining. It is also not uncommon to find iron up to 20 or even 30 ppm in rural water.

Iron may occur in water as ferrous bicarbonate

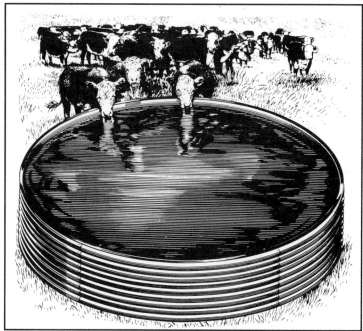

WATER IS CRITICAL. Some 60% to 85% of the daily nutrition needs of all farm animals is represented by water.

which, when dissolved, is colorless. However, as soon as the water is drawn and comes into contact with the air, the iron oxidizes and becomes the insoluble ferric hydroxide. This oxidation causes the familiar reddish discoloration in water. Carbon dioxide is a by-product of this process.

Oxidation (hypochlorite), precipitation and filtering are the methods of removal with filtering being the most economical method of treatment. Iron carried in water may be removed by getting rid of the acid condition and filtering.

Acid may be removed by aeration. Passing the water over crushed limestone will remove much of the carbon dioxide which is responsible for holding the iron in suspension. Sometimes, treatment with chlorine will remove some iron.

Manganese

Often, manganese accompanies iron and reacts similarly, leaving a black stain. Removal is the same as outlined for iron.

Hydrogen Sulfide

Generally found in deep wells, this compound in large amounts can be poisonous. As little as 1 ppm will produce an objectionable smell. This gas is a weak acid which eventually attacks the iron, forming iron sulfide. These deposits are black and feel greasy.

Hydrogen sulfide can be removed by oxidation or activated charcoal filtering. The most economical method is oxidation by a chemical such as hypochlorite. It will change the gas to elemental sulfur which can then be filtered.

Carbon Dioxide

Carbon dioxide is sometimes absorbed from the air, but many times it comes from the organic acids of decaying vegetable matter. It forms a carbonic acid which corrodes copper pipes. The addition of a buffering agent such as sodium carbonate or magnesia will neutralize the acid effect of carbon dioxide. Magnesia and/or limestone filters can be used to eliminate any carbon dioxide problems.

Pesticides And Herbicides

Activated charcoal filters are the treatment of choice for water contaminated with herbicides, pesticides, DDT, etc. However, when a well is contaminated with these chemicals, it is best to completely clean the well by flushing rather than relying on a single small filter to do the job of purification.

Other elements may also prove harmful if found in high concentrations. The Environmental Protection Agency (EPA) has established criteria for quality drinking water for livestock and poultry.

Besides these criteria, the EPA also lists the following points necessary for quality water:

- No heavy growths of blue-green algae.

- Amount of pesticides not to exceed limits prescribed for drinking water.

- Radionuclides not to exceed limits prescribed in federal drinking water standards.

- Salinity not to exceed 300 mg soluble salts per liter.

Suspect Contamination

Virtually all sources of water should be suspected of contamination. Surface water (ponds, streams, lakes) usually is lower in mineral content than ground water, but may be more heavily contaminated with bacteria. Ground water will usually have heavier concentrations of dissolved minerals than surface water, depending on the type of soil or rock through which it percolates.

Shallow wells are subject to leaching of contaminants. Deep wells depend on ground water and draw their water from a considerable distance and from different places during different times of the year. Therefore, it is important that water from these sources be spot-checked periodically.

Methods of water purification include water softening, filtering, precipitation, chlorination, reverse osmosis, ozone treatment, exposure to ultraviolet and/or ultrasonics, etc. While all these treatments have their specific benefits, the most common water treatments are softening, filtering and chlorination.

The primary use of water softeners is to remove hardness from the water. However, as previously mentioned, the concept that soft water is superior to hard water is not always valid. The minerals found in hard water can be quite beneficial if their levels are not excessively high. Increasing the sodium ion concentration to an abnormally high level can also be detrimental.

For instance, the following are typical water test analysis results:

Typical Water Analysis Results

Element Teste	Prior To Softening	Post Softening
Calcium	75 ppm	3.2 ppm
Sodium	34 ppm	270 ppm
Magnesium	20 ppm	.1 ppm
Potassium	19 ppm	8 ppm

Filtering and precipitation have the obvious limitations of selectivity. Reverse osmosis is still a relatively expensive process, although technologically very sound.

Besides softening, chlorination is probably the most widely used method of water purification. This is probably because bacteria pose a greater threat to the health and productivity of animals than dissolved ions. At the present time, chlorination is the treatment of choice when dealing with bacteria-contaminated water.

Proper Chlorination Is A Key

By properly chlorinating your water supply, you will be able to:

- Kill all pathogenic bacteria as long as residual chlorine remains in the water.

- Kill slime through oxidation.

- Convert iron to particle form, facilitating filtering and preventing oxidizing of surfaces (rust).

- Eliminate rotten egg odor and sulfur corrosion.

- Oxidize manganese and present its oxidation on equipment.

- Kill iron bacteria through oxidation.

From this list, it is obvious that chlorine's action is largely a result of its oxidizing capability. Chlorine and water form hypochlorous acid which provides the needed active oxygen for oxidation.

Chlorine As A Disinfectant

Six important factors determine the effectiveness of chlorine as a disinfectant:

☛ *Type and Concentration of Chlorine:* Chlorination with "free" chlorine residuals is much more effective than with "combined or chloramine" residuals. With either free or combined chlorine residuals, disinfection becomes more effective with increasing residuals.

☛ *There are three basic sources of chlorine on the market today:* chlorine gas, calcium hypochlorite (70% chlorine) and sodium hypochlorite (5% chlorine).

☛ *pH of Water:* Disinfection of water with chlorine is significantly more effective at low pH values (6 to 7) than at higher pH values (9 to 10).

☛ *Duration of Organisms' Contact with Chlorine:* With both free and combined chlorine residuals, the effectiveness of disinfection increases with the time of contact.

☛ *Temperature of Water:* With both free and combined chlorine residuals, effectiveness of disinfection is boosted with increases of temperature within the normal water temperature range.

☛ *Types of Organisms Present:* Different microorganisms react differently under various combinations of factors, determining the effectiveness of disinfection with chlorine.

United States Public Health Service (USPHS) Drinking Water Standards

Chemical	USPHS Limit Not To Exceed
Nitrates	45 ppm
Nitrites*	.03 ppm
Iron	.3 ppm
Hardness*	0-3 GPG (soft) 4 GPG—on up (hard)
Phosphate*	5 ppm (denotes sewage)
Precipitation	Not applicable
Sulfate	250 ppm
Hydrogen sulfide	.1 ppm
pH	7—neutral
Arsenic	.01 ppm
Chlorine	Not applicable
Copper	1 ppm
Cyanide	.01 ppm
Fluoride	.7-1.2 ppm
Zinc	5 ppm
Silver	.05 ppm
Selenium	.01 ppm
Manganese	.05 ppm
Lead	.05 ppm

Limits accepted by most laboratories

☞ *Chlorine Demand of the Water:* An increase in the chlorine demand of the water increases the

```
┌─────────────────────────────────────────┐
│                                           │
│      USPHS Bacteriologic Standards        │
│           For Water Supplies              │
│                                           │
│   Satisfactory      Coliform bacteria     │
│                     (M.P.N)—0             │
│                                           │
│   Unsatisfactory    Coliform bacteria     │
│                     (M.P.N.)—1to 8        │
│                                           │
│   Unsafe            Coliform bacteria     │
│                     (M.P.N.)-9 or more    │
│                                           │
└─────────────────────────────────────────┘
```

amount of chlorine required to obtain a satisfactory free chlorine residual.

Superchlorination Works

Because of the duration of an organism's contact with chlorine, an improved method of chlorination has been developed to increase effectiveness and decrease needed exposure time. This method is termed "Superchlorination."

"Superchlorination" must be used as the correct term to describe the system in order to differentiate it from the "chlorination" systems used in municipal water plants. The latter process involves holding quite low concentrations of chlorine in water for a long period of time.

Superchlorination is just the opposite—a relatively large amount of chlorine is used, but the time is quite short.

Valuable Reference Facts About Water Measures

1 gal. equals 4 qts.

1 cubic foot equals 7.48 gal. of water.

1 gal. of water weighs approximately 8.33 lbs.

1 gal. of milk weighs approximately 8.6 lbs.

1 liter equals approximately 1.057 qts.

1 liter equals .2642 gal.

1 gallon equals 3.785 liters.

1 part per million (ppm) equals 1 miligram (mg) per liter.

1 ppm equals 1 gram per cubic meter.

1 ppm equals 0.058 grains per gallon.

1 grain per gallon equals 17.1 ppm.

1 grain per gallon equals 17.1 mg per liter.

1 grain equals 1/7000 lb.

Superchlorination is actually a far more effective, more efficient way of treating water. However, it might take humans some additional time to become adjusted to the chlorine taste. This apparently isn't a great problem with livestock.

Tests at John Hopkins Univ. revealed that in the presence of 10 ppm of free available chlorine (water pH below 8.0, temperature of 4.0 C) 90% of the tested E. coli population was killed within 0.7 seconds and 99% within 1.5 seconds. No surviving E. coli from test population in the range of 25,000 to 125,000 per 100 ml could be obtained in samples where 10 ppm free chlorine residuals existed for 5.0 seconds or more.

However, there are some water quality problems that superchlorination will not overcome. It will not soften hard water. It will not remove nitrates nor will it remove salty or alkali tastes. Likewise, superchlorination will not remove rare chemicals such as selenium, lead, arsenic, etc.

The obvious pitfall of thinking of superchlorination as a panacea for all livestock water problems must be avoided. It is not, nor are other water purification methods, a substitute for the repair of a faulty water supply. Every effort should be made to remove the source of the contamination.

Superchlorination can be an insurance policy against disease losses via the water supply. If properly used, it is a safe, sound, and economical method of water purification. As with all water purification methods, superchlorination should be implemented only on the advice of qualified professionals in the water quality field.

Using A Balling Gun

A GOOD balling gun simplifies giving capsules or boluses to cattle, sheep, swine, goats or horses. Its use is one of the oldest methods for getting pills and capsules into the stomach of an animal.

Results from putting medicines into the stomach are slower than intravenous medication. These drugs must be absorbed from the digestive tract before they will get into the blood stream to act on other parts of the body.

A balling gun is a simple device with a hollow head

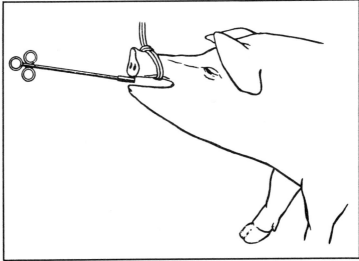

BALLING GUN USAGE. To handle a grown hog for veterinary treatment with a balling gun, tie and hold the animal as shown here. Follow the detailed instructions found in this article for placing all pills or boluses in the hog's mouth.

which holds the capsule or bolus until dislodged with a plunger.

As in drenching, some type of restraint is often necessary with large, unruly animals. However, most animals can be held with a nose lead or rope on halter around the neck. Directions on how to properly use a restraint can be found in the next chapter on drenching livestock.

Balling Gun

Administering pills or boluses to hogs is especially difficult because the odd shape of the back of the throat forms a pocket where the hog can lodge and hold a pill to be spit out later. After treating hogs, watch them closely to see if they drop or cough up the pill or bolus. It is helpful to treat pigs in a pen

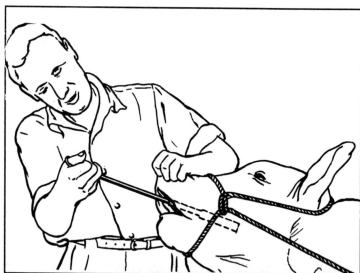

HOW IT IS EASILY DONE. This drawing shows how to hold a cow and administer a pill or bolus with the balling gun. Note how far the balling gun is inserted into the mouth.

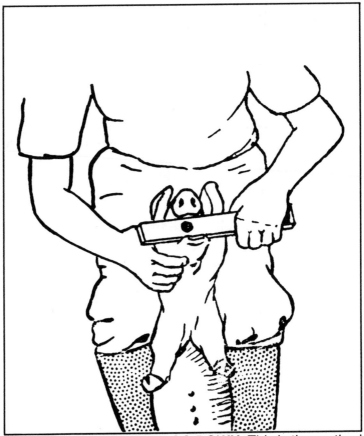

MAKING THE MEDICINE GO DOWN. This is the method for holding a small pig and using a homemade gag to administer medicine by balling gun or with a dose syringe.

with a bare, clean floor where the bolus can be found if expelled by the animal.

Follow these all-important steps to give medicine with a balling gun:

☞ Place the capsule or bolus in the head of the "gun."

☞ Hold or restrain the animal as necessary. The

head is best held steady with the left arm over the bridge of the nose.

☞ The capsule should be placed in the animal's mouth well back over the middle of the base of the tongue. It should be dropped by the plunger action so it is automatically swallowed by reflex action of the throat muscles. It is released from the gun by pressing the plunger. If any coughing or choking occurs, free the head at once so the animal can lower it to "cough out" the cause. You have to use care so the capsule goes into the gullet—not the windpipe— to prevent its lodging in the throat.

From following these basic steps, it is easy to see that using a balling gun is quite simple. In addition to the balling gun, balling irons and capsule forceps are sometimes also used.

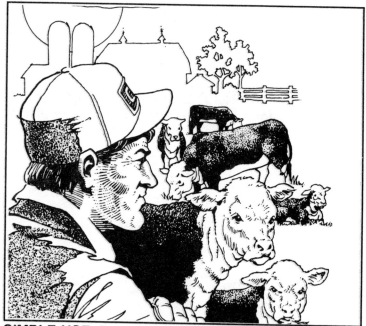

SIMPLE USE. Based on the simple steps outlined here, you can see using a balling gun is a very easy operation.

Balling Irons

A balling iron or mouth speculum is a device which can be placed in the mouth as a jaw spreader to aid in giving capsules with the use of a balling gun or capsule forceps. In addition to spreading the jaws, the balling iron helps hold the jaw open as well as hold the animal still. The balling gun and its capsule is placed in the mouth through the balling iron and the capsule is dropped to the rear of the tongue.

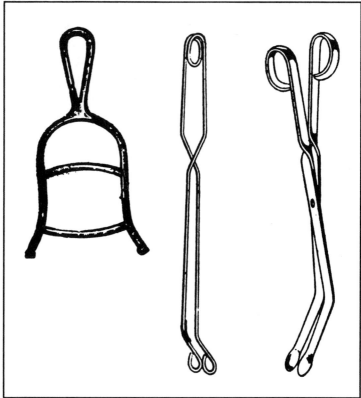

BALLING GUN ACCESSORIES. A balling iron or mouth speculum and two types of balling forceps are shown her The bolus or pill is held between the jaws of the forceps and is easily and safely dropped into the animal's mouth.

Balling irons are especially useful in administering capsules to hogs, sheep and other small animals. They are used much less frequently with larger animals such as cattle and horses.

Capsule Forceps

Capsule forceps are somewhat similar to a balling gun except they hold the capsule securely between two jaws. Placed into the animal's mouth, the capsule is dropped instead of being forced out by a plunger as in a gun.

Capsule forceps are usually used with a balling iron and are most often used with smaller animals such as swine, sheep or goats. Their only advantage is that they are cheaper than a balling gun. However, they do not place the medicine capsule "into the gullet" as well as a balling gun.

Chapter 11

Practical Ideas For Drenching Livestock

PROBABLY THE simplest way of administering medicine to livestock is to mix it in their feed or drinking water. But this won't always work, especially if the medicine has a disagreeable taste or odor. The medicine in such cases can be poured down the animal's throat into the stomach by means of a rubber tube or into its mouth from a long-necked bottle by drenching.

How It Works

Drenching must be performed very carefully or part of the liquid may go into the animal's lung. This can cause gangrene or pneumonia and result in death.

The entrance to the animal's gullet is closed by a "valve" except when the animal is in the act of swallowing. The entrance to the windpipe remains open while an animal is breathing normally. However, it has to close when the animal swallows.

When medicine is poured into the animal's throat and the animal does not swallow voluntarily, medicine will go down the windpipe instead of the gullet. The liquid then enters the lungs instead of the stomach for which it was intended.

Unfortunately, an oil drenching solution is an especially dangerous liquid to use. It will not evaporate like water when it goes into the wrong place.

Although drenching is somewhat hazardous, it can be performed safely if ordinary precautions are taken.

Restraint Is Helpful

The job of drenching is made much easier if a simple homemade restraint is used. This is particularly important with larger animals like cattle and horses.

A light rope or sash cord, about 8 ft. long, should be doubled in the middle. The ends of the rope are then passed through the resulting loop to form a noose. This noose is slipped over the animal's upper jaw, working it well back into the mouth and drawing it tight.

After the noose is placed and the drench prepared as described in the following paragraphs, the head can be raise slightly—just enough so the medicine in the mouth will flow toward the throat. Fasten the rope in position by tying the ends of it to the stanchion top or other sturdy object. Be sure to tie the rope so it can be released quickly as described later on.

If the head is raised too high, the danger of strangling the animal is greatly increased. You can hold the head in the right position by grasping the nostrils between the thumb and forefinger.

Besides immobilizing the head, the rope restraint in the animal's mouth forces it to keep the mouth open and make constant chewing movements. This helps the animal swallow the medicine with much less danger of breathing it into the lungs.

Some livestock producers find a nose lead works well for raising the head and restraining livestock while they are being drenched. This is quite practical if one is available at the time of drenching.

Use A Drenching Bottle

It is wise to keep a special bottle for drenching in your livestock medicine chest. An ordinary quart size long-necked bottle may be used with a short piece of rubber hose used to extend the neck of the bottle. The added length allows liquids to be placed well back in the mouth so they are sure to be swallowed. At the same time, it avoids the danger of the bottle neck being broken off between the animal's teeth.

Drenching bottles made of plastic and with a long rubber nozzle are also available. They are safer and easier to use and the cost is small.

Metal and plastic drenching syringes are also available. Their use is similar to using a bottle except a plunger or "piston" inside a metal cylinder forces the liquid out. Never attempt to forcefully spray liquid with a syringe. Slowly push the plunger down to allow the liquid to flow at the rate an animal is able to swallow.

Measure all medicines that go into the drenching solution carefully. Never guess at the quantity. Too much may be harmful and can even lead to death.

How To Drench

After the drenching solution has been carefully prepared, placed in the bottle or syringe and the animal securely held or restrained, follow these steps:

☛ Elevate the animal's nose until it forms a straight line with the neck. If the head is held too high, such a position interferes with swallowing and increases the danger of allowing the mixture to get into the lungs. The animal's head is best held steady with your left arm over the bridge of the nose.

☛ The neck of the drenching bottle should be put

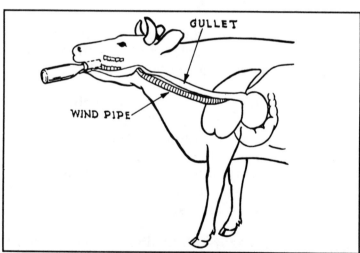

HOW TO DO IT. To drench, use a long bottle with a rubber tube over the tip. Lift the animal's head just above normal, keeping the neck straight. Insert the drenching bottle or dose syringe in the right corner of the animal's mouth, bringing the top of the bottle or the end of its rubber tube extension so that it is left directly in front of the back teeth.

into the side of the animal's mouth so the open tip of the bottle or tube rests along the middle of the tongue. Care should be taken to avoid getting the bottle between the teeth (especially those in the back of the mouth) as the bottle could be broken. The medicine will flow slowly and naturally in this position.

☞ Never give too much liquid at a time. A drench of 2 oz. is plenty with cattle and other large animals. Use even less with smaller livestock such as sheep. Allow about 1 minute for swallowing the solution and breathing before giving the next dose. The medicine should be poured slowly while the mouth is closed. If the animal coughs, the head should be lowered at once to permit the fluid to escape.

Several other drenching hints which you can put to good use include the following:

- Always free the head whenever coughing starts so it can be lowered to help the animal free any liquid which might enter the lungs.

- Never pull the tongue out of the mouth since it needs to be free to aid in the natural reflex of swallowing.

- Whenever more than 1 pt. of liquid must be given as a drench, allow 10 or 15 minutes' rest between doses.

- Clean your drenching bottle or syringe well after each use. It will then be in good condition for its next use.

- Drenching animals when they have milk fever or there is paralysis of the throat due to other causes is dangerous and usually fatal. Great care also must be exercised when drenching animals that are lying down. Drenching usually results in death when treating bloat that is caused by choking. Be sure there is no paralysis of the throat or plugging of the esophagus.

- Sheep generally are more difficult to drench than cows. Never drench sheep unless you have them standing firmly on all four feet. Never raise their noses any higher than their eyes during the drenching process. Sheep are often given medicines with a syringe or through a piece of rubber tubing with a funnel attached to one end and a metal tube to the other end. The metal tube is carefully inserted into the sheep's gullet and the medicine is poured slowly into the funnel.

By carefully following these time-tested directions you can safely and easily administer a variety of drench materials to your livestock.

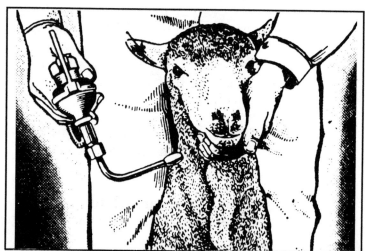

EASY SHEEP DRENCHING. Several types of special drench guns are used for large scale drenching of flocks of sheep. A large supply of drench medicine is contained in a storage bag and then can be released automatically.

Chapter 12

Castrating With An Emasculatome

THE EMASCULATOME (Burdizzo pincer) is a precision made instrument for the humane, bloodless castration of livestock having a pendulous scrotum. It operates as a dull pincher or clamp to crush and sever the testicular cord without greatly injuring the bag or scrotum.

There is no open wound and therefore little danger of loss from blood poisoning, flies or screw worms. Deprived of nourishing blood, the testicles immediately stop the production of seminal fluid and wither away in about 6 weeks.

One problem with older types of esmasculatomes-the slipping of the testicular cord from between the jaws—is now prevented by "cordstop", metal protrusions on the jaws of the instrument. The cord is held in place without assistance and slipping of the cord is almost impossible if directions are carefully followed.

Needless to say, the livestock producer must be careful to follow all instructions. Careless use of the instrument may result in many partly castrated animals.

A number of different emasculatomes are manufactured. These include a 9 in. long baby unit, 12 in. small size for rams, calves and docking of lamb tails, 13 in. medium size for rams and calves, 16 in.

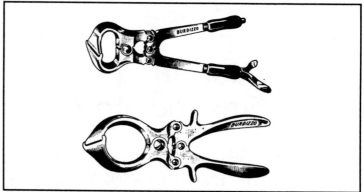

TWO TYPES OF EMASCULATOMES. The larger instrument shown at the top is fitted with a knee rest to facilitate operating on cattle. The smaller instrument shown at the bottom is 9 in. long. Note cordstops at the sides of the jaws.

large size for bulls and colts and the 19 in. indian size for bulls and horses.

Preventing Wounds

Other methods of castration produce a wound which exposes the animal to infestation from screw wounds. The emasculatome does not produce a large open wound as the greater part of the skin of the scrotum is kept intact so blood may circulate normally. No flies are attracted and blow-fly complications are next to impossible.

Castration with this method can be done year round regardless of the presence or absence of flies. With a little smear of pinetrol, it is practically fly-proof in warm weather.

Cattle and sheep castrated with this tool feel little shock and are not set back in condition or thrown off feed. There is consequently no season or weather condition that may prevent stockowners from operating. No special attention or treatment other than free exercise is necessary after the operation.

Castrating Lambs

The two most proper methods of castrating male sheep are by the knife and by the bloodless castrator. There are various minor modifications with the knife method, but the essential fact is that both testicles are removed, unless one or both have not descended. With bloodless castration, the spermatic cord is crushed and the testicle slowly degenerates (complete atrophy). It has been claimed the degenerating testicle stimulates growth, resulting in a better grown wether at sale time.

Correct use of the emasculatome is a matter of patience and acquired skill. It is better to castrate when lambs have reached a fair size and their testicles are fully descended. It is also advisable to have two men handle the job, one to hold the lamb and the second to work the instrument.

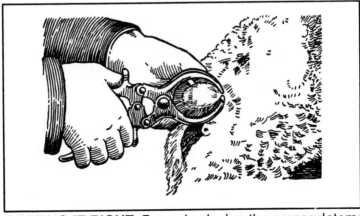

GETTING IT RIGHT. Properly placing the emasculatome prior to starting to operate on a male lamb is very critical.

Emasculatomes without a cordstop require a third man to pull down the testicle and steady the cord.

Here are the steps to follow in successfully using this type of instrument:

☛ Lambs must be held by an assistant. Have him stand facing the operator and on the opposite side of a small table. Grasping each lamb by the front legs, he swings the animal onto the table holding the front feet high so the lamb's rump rests on the table in a sitting position. The back legs are spread, presenting the scrotum conveniently to the operator.

☛ The operator grasps the bag or scrotum with the left hand and with thumb and finger forces the left testicular cord against the left side of the bag. The tool is held open with the right hand, taking care that the jaw with the cordstop is the lower one.

☛ The jaws of the emasculatome are placed with the right hand over the skin of the bag, taking in the left projecting cord so the cord is resting just inside the cordstop projection.

☛ In this way, the thumb of the left hand should feel the cordstop through the skin of the bag and exert a slight pressure against it. Now clamp the tool quickly and fully onto the cord.

☛ The thumb and second finger of the left hand are slid forward slightly, pressing the cord close to the jaws of the instrument until the cord gives way. This indicates it has been completely severed. The tool is then quickly released and the same procedure is repeated on the right testicular cord.

Castrating Rams

With an assistant grasping the front feet and holding the ram in sitting position on a small table or box, the operator grasps the scrotum and with his left hand holds one testicular cord in place.

With the emasculatome open and held by the upper handle, it is swung into place by the right hand. With the lower handle resting on the table top, the upper handle is pressed down until the pincers are fully closed.

The operator then fully severs the cord with his fingers and proceeds to perform the same operation on the remaining testicular cord.

Docking Lambs' Tails

To remove lamb tails, close the 12 in. tool on the tail between the first and second bone. Cut the tail

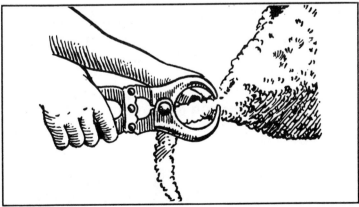

QUICK AND EASY. One big benefit of using this method of docking tails in a sheep flock is that it prevents bleeding.

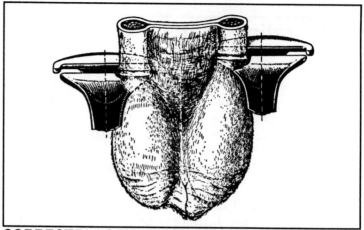

CORRECT PLACEMENT IS CRITICAL. The way in which an emasculatome easily crushes the testicular cords without cutting the scrotum of the animal is clearly shown here. Note the correct placement of the instrument on both sides.

off inside the closed jaws, then treat the cut with pinetrol or some other similar fly repellent and release the lamb. The crush of the pincers should prevent bleeding.

Using With Cattle

The use of this instrument on calves is a simple, safe and bloodless operation if a number of step-by-step instructions are carefully followed.

Tie the calf to a manger or post as short as possible to restrain its movements. With the animal standing, have an assistant push it against the manger or wall.

The assistant should raise the end of the animal's tail and bend it back over the spine. This will prevent the calf from kicking. Do not tie the legs because it only further irritates the animal. Handle the testicles as little as possible as it makes the calf uneasy. Follow these steps:

☞ The bull calf is castrated in a standing position. Stand behind the animal, holding the instrument open with the right hand.

☞ With the fingers of the left hand, feel for and close on the cord of the left testicle pushing it against the lateral wall of the bag. With the right hand, place the jaws of the tool on the cord.

☞ With the help of the right knee, close the pincers until the cord is compressed enough to be held in place. Care must be taken so the cord does not slip out. A special knee rest is supplied with

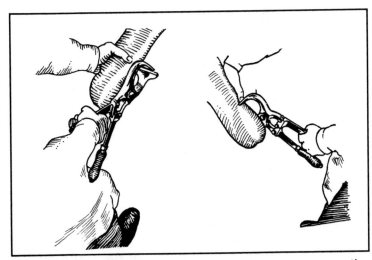

KNEE REST HELPS. With the knee rest accessory on the emasculatome shown at left, the lower handle of the instrument rests on the right knee until the operator makes certain the cord is in the right place for crushing. At right, with the emasculatome closed, feel for the cord above the jaws with your thumb and forefinger until your fingers almost meet. This indicates the cord is completely severed.

some emasculatomes and can be used to help close the pincers with the right knee.

☛ Apply both hands on the wooden handles of the pincers and press firmly until the instrument is completely closed. Care must be taken so the cord does not slip out of place in the pincers.

☛ To make sure the cord is crushed, press on the cord immediately above the jaws of the pincers with your thumb and second finger until these fingers almost meet. This indicates the cord is completely severed.

☛ Repeat the operation on the cord of the right testicle and the bull is castrated.

Two minutes should be sufficient time to complete the operation. Immediately after the blood vessels of the cord are crushed, the flow of blood to the testicles is stopped. Complete atrophy is noticed about 40 days after the operation without the animal suffering or requiring any special treatment or attention.

When old bulls or horses are castrated with this method, the cord can be better held under the crush of the tool by means of a pair of slightly modified pliers.

In summary, the emasculatome or Burdizzo pincers are a valuable farm veterinary instrument. They cause little or no setback. They are much more humane than using a knife. No blood is lost and they prevent infections because the scrotum isn't cut.

Chapter 13

Controlling Internal Parasites In Your Cattle

SHOULD I worm my cattle? What wormer should I use? How can I tell if my cattle are wormy? Where is the economic point in worming? Will worming pay?

These are some of the questions that have been typically asked by cattlemen—both beef and dairy producers—for many years. And they are still asking the same questions.

Internal parasitism in cattle is a problem with many variables which does not lend itself to one specific type of recommendation. Consequently, the questions are still coming and many are still unanswerable.

Economic Returns For Worming

There is ample material found in the literature dealing with types of parasites, their life cycles and identification. Information is also available on the economic return when using chemicals to control internal infections.

Most surveys show all ruminants to be parasitized to some extent—if fecal examinations are used as the criteria to determine parasitism. Variables affecting a diagnosis are the type of internal parasite and its egg-laying abilities, arrested state of ingested larvae, differentiation of type of internal parasite and the environmental conditions under which the host exists.

Most studies show that roughly 90% of all cattle are sustaining some sort of an economic loss.

Tough To Measure

The way parasites affect their hosts is not always measurable. It is difficult to measure the factors individually such as the way parasites affect their host's tissues, how they affect nutrient absorption, the effect on the host's body fluids, possible mechanical damage to internal organs and the portals of entry which internal parasites can cause for pathogenic bacteria. Feed efficiency and rate of gain are often the only criterion used to determine the economics of using internal parasite control in cattle. However, other factors must also be considered.

Environmental factors are rapidly changing. Concentration of animals in confined areas tends to also increase the parasite load. However, in confinement systems with the use of slotted floors, recontamination of animals is limited.

In general, a review of most studies shows internal parasites reduce the overall productivity of most cattle by 5% to 10%.

Diagnosis Of Internal Parasites

Historically, fecal examinations have been used to determine the level of internal parasitism. The type of internal parasite and the stage of the cycle will affect the numbers of eggs.

Eggs per gram of feces is not a reliable criterion to determine the economic level of treatment. Clinical appearance and hematocrits (packed red blood cell volume) may be used. However, most feeding trials show a low level of parasitism will affect feed efficiency. This could not be determined by fecal examination and clinical pathology.

Prevention And Control

The age of the animal, its environment and level of nutrition all affect the level of parasitism in ruminants. The concept of preventing recontamination has not been taught as an animal practice.

The practices of keeping all ages of cattle together, feeding hay off the ground and failure to use anthelmintics routinely have contributed to parasitism in many herds. The choice of the best anthelmintic for control depends upon whether you prefer to drench, administer a bolus, incorporate it into feed or inject it into the animal's body.

Your veterinarian can assist you in the selection and administration of the wormer.

In Review

Remember these key points when working out a program for battling internal parasites in cattle:

1 Most ruminant animals will be parasitized to some extent.

2 Fecal determinations are not always easily made and diagnosed.

3 Anthelmintics now on the market are efficacious.

4 Systems of animal husbandry need to be changed.

5 Strategic deworming programs are recommended.

In view of the present systems being used by livestock producers and soaring costs for producing meat and milk, it appears to be a very sound practice to properly control internal parasites.

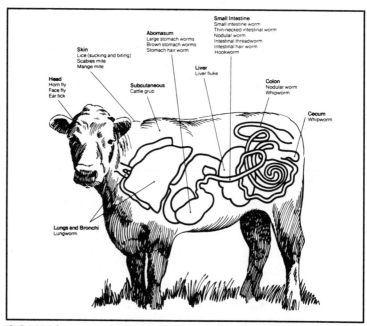

Small Intestine
Small intestine worm
Thin-necked intestinal worm
Nodular worm
Intestinal threadworm
Intestinal hair worm
Hookworm

Abomasum
Large stomach worms
Brown stomach worms
Stomach hair worm

Skin
Lice (sucking and biting)
Scabies mite
Mange mite

Liver
Liver fluke

Head
Horn fly
Face fly
Ear tick

Subcutaneous
Cattle grub

Colon
Nodular worm
Whipworm

Cecum
Whipworm

Lungs and Bronchi
Lungworm

COMMON PARASITES OF CATTLE. This diagram shows the common internal and external parasites of cattle in the United States and the organs they attack. Not all parasites are found in every area, but each cattle-production area harbors several internal and external parasites.

Chapter 14

Bloat Prevention
And Treatment

BLOAT IS A form of indigestion marked by an abnormal collection of gas in the rumen. Bloat results when the animal is not able to eructate or belch the large volume of gases produced during rumen fermentation.

Several contributing causes of bloat include: an inherited tendency for bloat, certain proteins in forage, the amount and rate of roughage intake, the coarseness of the roughage, the rumen microbial population and enlargement of the lymph nodes between the lungs which compress the esophagus or interfere with the function of the vagus nerves (following respiratory infection, diagnosis can only be confirmed during necropsy).

Basically, there are two kinds of bloat—pasture bloat and feedlot bloat.

Pasture bloat usually occurs in animals grazing lush alfalfa (or other legumes such as ladino or red clover) or fed green-chopped legumes in the feedlot.

Feedlot bloat usually refers to bloat in cattle being fed high grain rations which may or may not contain legume forages. Because of the complex causes, different methods of preventing bloat must be used.

Preventing Pasture Bloat

Many methods have been used over the years to reduce the incidence of pasture bloat. Poloxalene is an anti-foaming agent which prevents pasture bloat for 12 hours if fed in adequate amounts. Poloxalene can be fed as a top dressing on feed, in a grain mixture fed free choice or in molasses-salt blocks. The problem with each of these methods is insuring that every animal gets an adequate intake of Poloxalene each day to prevent bloat.

The cost of bloat prevention using Poloxalene is 5 to 8 cents per head daily. Some livestock producers consider this rather expensive compared to the risk in many pastures. In addition, it is difficult at times to get the correct intake of Poloxalene at the right time to completely prevent bloat. Relying on methods of management to reduce bloat danger may be justified even when Poloxalene is being fed.

A fairly new bloat preventative known as Bloat Blox, which contains Laureth-23, has also been found to be effective in controlling bloat in cattle.

To help reduce the occurrence of bloat, try following these time-tested practical management ideas:

1 Plant and manage pastures to contain no more than 50% alfalfa forage.

2 Fill cattle up on dry roughage or grass pasture before turning them into legume pastures.

3 Feed dry hay or mow a few strips and leave the forage in the field as a source of dry roughage.

4 Provide a choice of grass pasture along with the legume pasture.

5 Feed grain or a grain-roughage mixture to reduce pasture intake. If Poloxalene is hand-fed on top of a small amount of feed once or twice daily, plan the time of feeding to give the greatest possible protection following heavy intake of legume forage which usually occurs in early morning and late evening.

6 Do not turn cattle out on a pasture which is wet with dew or rain.

7 Once your cattle are turned out into a pasture, don't remove them at the first signs of bloat. Mild subacute bloat occurs frequently and repeatedly on alfalfa pasture. When cattle are first turned into a pasture, leave them until the rumen is greatly distended or until the first signs of distress from bloat appears. Then remove only the bloated cattle if just a small percentage of the cattle are affected.

8 When feeding green chop, spread forage intake over the whole day. This can be done by feeding several times daily or by full feeding the green-chop mixed with a substantial amount of grain.

Managing Feedlot Bloat

Feedlot bloat occurs infrequently and death losses are normally minimal in well-managed feedlots.

Most cases are subacute rather than acute where distress symptoms such as frequent urination and defecation, labored breathing and restless movements are evident. Feedlot bloat is quite often of a chronic nature, occurring repeatedly in only a few of the cattle found in a particular lot.

Under these conditions, Poloxalene does not appear to be effective in preventing feedlot bloat even though rumen foam is often involved.

The ration most commonly fed by feeders seeking information regarding control of feedlot bloat has included finely ground grain and loose alfalfa hay fed in separate bunks or finely chopped alfalfa hay mixed with grain.

Using these rations as a basis for discussion, the following ideas may prove effective in reducing the frequency and severity of bloat—offered in the approximate order of preference:

☞ Coarse chop hay and mix with the grain.

☞ Increase the amount of hay fed to 15% of the ration dry matter.

☞ Use a coarser roll on the grain.

☞ Substitute low quality legume or non-legume roughage for part or all of the alfalfa hay (adjust the protein, vitamin and mineral supplement appropriately as needed at the same time).

☞ Feed 50% or more coarsely rolled corn or whole corn.

Feedlot bloat which occurs when feeding high concentrate or all-concentrate rations can usually be reduced by adding coarsely chopped roughage to bring the roughage content to 10% to 15% of the total ration. In some cases separation of the grain from roughage and/or supplement seems to be involved. When this is a problem, change the ration to minimize separation.

Bloat Treatment

Acute bloat must be treated promptly if death is to be avoided. In the last stages of severe bloat, even a few seconds delay may result in death.

Plan well in advance with your veterinarian for possible emergency treatment for bloat ahead of

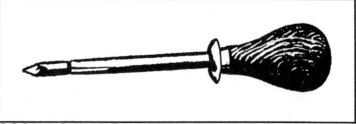

GOOD INSURANCE. While having a trocar is good insurance, using one is likely to cause a dangerous infection even when the animal survives. As a last resort for controlling bloat, keep one of these items on hand and know how to use it. The trocar shown here is encased in its cannula, which is the part that remains within the animal's loin to allow problem gas to escape after the trocar is withdrawn.

the upcoming pasture season. You'll need:

- Good handling facilities.

- A 3/4 in. to 1 in. diameter rubber hose that is and 8 to 10 ft. long.

- A supply of defoaming agent—in an emergency, household detergents can be used; mix a cupful in 5 gal. of water.

- A large trocar (and a sharp knife suitable for opening an incision into the rumen if the trocar

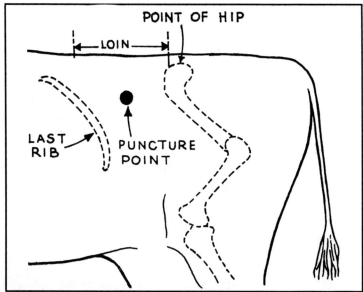

PUNCTURE POINTS. These marks show the approximate position where a bloated cow should be tapped with a trocar. The proper spot is along the left side as you stand behind her facing in the very same direction as the cow.

The location is about halfway between the last rib and the hipbone and a little more than 2 in. below the loin edge. The incision should be made at the place where there is the greatest extension of a bloated stomach. Be sure to keep in mind that a trocar should be used only after every other possible method of controlling the bloat has failed.

fails to relieve the bloat).

In addition, you'll need to know how to use the hose and antifoaming agent and to puncture the rumen if you are to be successful in bloat treatment.

In severe cases, the tube should be used to provide relief. This may not be enough with pasture bloat. If the tube does not provide immediate relief, the defoaming agent will frequently break the foam and permit removal of large amounts of gas through the tube or by the animal's belching. The antifoaming agent can be added either through the tube or by intraruminal injection.

Never attempt to drench a bloated animal. Drenching is likely to result in inhalation causing immediate death or pneumonia.

As a last resort, open a hole in the rumen large enough to release the foamy rumen contents. Insert the trocar at a point half-way between the last rib and hookbone or hipbone on the left side some 3 to 4 in. from the edge of the loin.

If the foam is so viscous than the trocar opening is not large enough to give relief, use a knife to open a slit about 2 in. long and spread it apart with your fingers. Keep at least one finger through the incision until the bloat is fully relieved. Otherwise, the rumen may move causing the opening in the rumen to shift away from the opening through the belly wall and skin.

Large bloat needles may be adequate for relieving feedlot bloat. These needles are 6 to 7 in. long and are supplied with a wire stylet with which to unplug them if necessary. They should be inserted high on the left side of the animal as indicated for use of the trocar in pasture bloat.

Chronic Bloat

Caused by enlargement of the lymph nodes between the lungs, this can be treated by making a rumen fistula. This procedure consists of making an opening through the skin and muscle high in the left flank. The rumen is then sutured to the skin before it is opened to release the accumulated gas. The fistula is designed to remain open for 1 or 2 months. During this time the lymph nodes should decrease in size and normal belching can resume. Normally, natural healing will close the fistula. If not, your veterinarian can surgically repair the opening.

Perhaps the best way to eliminate problems from chronic bloaters is to send these affected animals to slaughter, particularly if they weigh 700 lbs. or more.

Chapter 15

Properly Recognizing, Aiding Normal Calving

EXTRA CARE at calving time may certainly save a calf for future production in your herd.

If at all possible, be there when the cow calves. Leave her alone, but be nearby just in case the birth is not a normal one. When the cow is in serious trouble, be sure to call your veterinarian.

The first step, of course, is to have accurate breeding records. You should know when the cow will be ready to calve and watch for calving signs.

When she is due, get her into a box stall with plenty of clean dry bedding. Straw is best. If the weather is warm and you don't have a clean stall, put her in a pasture separated from the other cows.

Signs Of Early Calving

The first sign of calving, of course, is the making up of the udder or bagging which may begin as much as 4 to 6 weeks before the calf is born. Other distinguishing signs nearer calving the date will also show when a cow is due.

The cow shows increasing restlessness, moving around and mooing. The vulva becomes enlarged, congested and flabby. The pelvic ligaments relax and the area between the tailhead and pin bones is so loose and sunken that a fist can often be placed in each hollow.

There is spasmodic straining and the cow walks with difficulty, often looking at her own flank. Some 12 to 24 hours before birth, the cow's temperature will usually drop 1 or 2 degrees below normal. This is a sure sign the cow is ready to calve.

Just before actual calving begins, the water bladder appears and breaks. Soon afterwards, the calf's nose or foot follows, then two feet, the whole head and the shoulders. Once the shoulders (the broadest part) are through the passage, there is rarely any difficulty.

Drawing number one shows the appearance outside the vagina of the fetal membranes filled with fluid (water bag or bladder). Do not burst the water

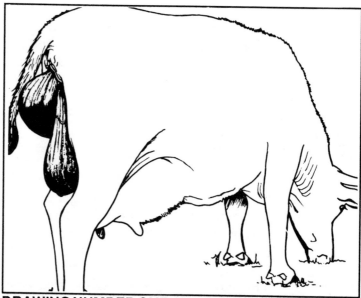

DRAWING NUMBER ONE. Note fetal membranes outside the cow which are filled with fluid. Do not break this water bag unless you are really sure an animal needs assistance.

bag unless you are sure the cow needs assistance and that you can deliver the calf safely and alive in a short period of time.

The purpose of the water bag or bladder is to dilate the womb and passage and make things easier for the calf to be born. The fluid it contains also acts as a "shock absorber" for the calf and a lubricant for the parts.

Once the fluid in the bag escapes, the calf tends to breathe. Unless it is delivered quickly, it can choke or drown from inhaling fluid left in the womb.

Drawing number two shows a water bag which has burst naturally. The fluid has escaped and is followed by the appearance of the head and fore feet. Note the relationship of the head to the legs—with the chin of the calf actually resting in the region of

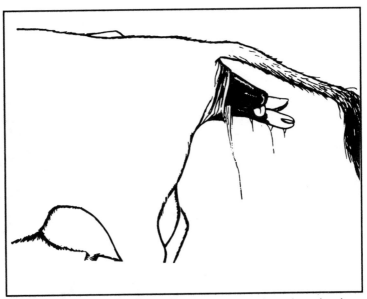

DRAWING NUMBER TWO. The water bag has broken naturally and the head and fore feet of the calf are now coming out. Note the relationship of the head to the legs.

the fetlock joints.

Remember this correct relationship when it is necessary for you to help the cow deliver her calf.

How, When To Assist

If the cow is calving naturally, do not assist her. Just make sure the nostrils and mouth of the calf are clear of mucus.

If a cow has been in labor 1 or 2 hours without delivering the calf, assistance is needed. A call to your veterinarian is your best bet. Don't let the cow labor too long or both the cow and calf may be lost.

Drawing number three shows the calf half deliv-

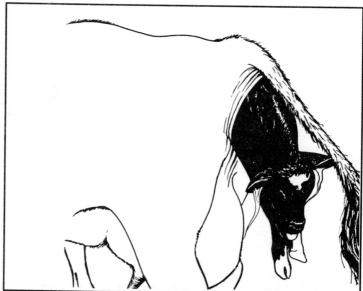

DRAWING NUMBER THREE. The calf is half delivered and the mouth and nose are clear. Any calf pulling should be in the same downward direction as shown by this calf.

ered; the nose and mouth are clear. This picture illustrates the correct direction in which traction must be applied, if it is necessary at all. The pull at this stage of delivery must be downward towards the hocks of the cow. This certainly reduces the risk of any obstruction occurring between the hips of the calf and the pelvis of the mother.

If some type of assistance is necessary, use clean nylon ropes attached to the calf's fetlocks to facilitate pulling. Nylon ropes are particularly useful since they can be more satisfactorily sterilized than hemp or manila ropes. Absolute cleanliness is very important. Traction or pull should be done in a downward motion as explained previously.

Drawing number four shows the calf safely delivered. In this case the umbilical cord attaching the calf to the fetal membranes has broken naturally.

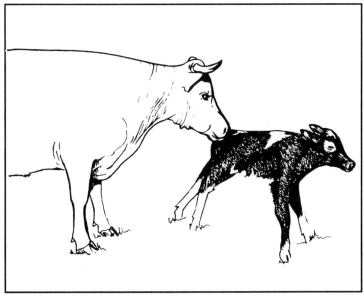

DRAWING NUMBER FOUR. The calf has now been safely delivered and the umbilical cord attaching the calf to the mother's fetal membranes has broken off naturally.

If the umbilical cord does not break naturally, a thin, but strong string soaked in tincture of iodine should be tied or ligatured around the cord about 2 in. from the calf's navel. Another string similarly prepared should be tied around the umbilical cord about 2 in. below the first string. Then cut the umbilical cord between the ligatures with a sharp knife.

Soak The Navel

It is a good idea to soak navels of all calves with tincture of iodine. This serves to prevent infection from contamination which may be present in a stall or pen.

A good licking by the mother is a fine stimulant to a new calf. Permit the cow to lick the calf immediately.

When the cow drops her tail into a normal position she generally has passed the afterbirth but this is not an infallible guide. If you are in doubt, remember that if is wise to recognize that more damage is done by removing afterbirth too soon than by leaving it. If needed, insert antiseptic uterine medication to prevent serious infection and decomposition on a daily basis.

Chapter 16

Making Injections In Your Cattle

BEFORE MAKING any kind of an injection, read the label carefully to determine product uses, cautions, proper dosage, frequency of administration and recommended methods of administration. Then consult the following directions for detailed instructions on how to make the type of injection which is recommended on the label.

Making An Intravenous Injection

An intravenous injection is made directly into the veins. This method is generally used when rapid and effective action is needed to save an animal's life.

Needed Equipment

- Choke rope—a rope or cord about 4 ft. long, with a loop in one end, to be used as a tourniquet.

- Gravity flow intravenous set.

- Hypodermic needles, 16 gauge, 1 1/2 in. long and very sharp. Use new needles as dull needles will not work. Extra needles should be available in case the one being used becomes clogged.

- Scissors or clippers.

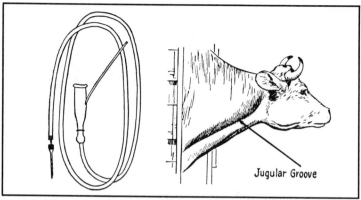

Jugular Groove

INTRAVENOUS EQUIPMENT. A gravity flow intravenous set is a necessary piece of equipment for any intravenous injections in cattle. This shows the proper location of the jugular groove which holds the vein for making an injection.

- 70% rubbing alcohol compound or an equally effective antiseptic for disinfecting the skin.

- The medication to be given.

Preparing Your Equipment

Thoroughly clean the needles and intravenous set and disinfect them by boiling in water for 20 minutes.

Warm the bottle of medication to approximately body temperature and keep warm until used.

Preparing Your Animals For Injection

Follow these steps to insure that the injections are made properly:

☛ Find the approximate location of the vein. The jugular vein runs in the groove on each side of the neck from the angle of the jaw to just above the brisket and slightly above and to the side of the windpipe.

☛ Some type of restraint—a stanchion or chute—is ideal for restraining the animal. With a halter, rope or cattle leader (nose tongs), pull the animal's head around the side of the stanchion, cattle chute or post in such a manner to form a bow in the neck. Snub the head securely to prevent movement.

☛ By forming a bow in the neck, the outside curvature of the bow tends to expose the jugular vein and make it easily accessible. Avoid a tight rope or halter around the throat or upper neck which might impede blood flow. Animals that are laying down present no problem as far as restraint is concerned.

☛ Clip the hair in the area where the injection is to be made (over the vein in the upper third of the neck). Clean and disinfect the skin with alcohol or other suitable antiseptic.

Entering The Vein And Injecting

Raise the vein by tying the choke rope tight around the neck, close to the shoulder. The rope should be tied in such a way that it will not come loose and can be untied quickly by pulling the loose end. In thick-necked animals, a block of wood placed in the jugular groove between the rope and the hide will help considerably in applying the desired pressure to the right point.

The vein is a soft flexible tube through which blood flows back to the heart. Under ordinary conditions, it cannot be seen or felt with the fingers. When the flow of blood is blocked at the base of the neck by

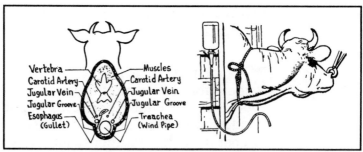

HOW TO FIND IT. This cross section of a beef or dairy animal's neck shows the location of the jugular vein in relation to other cattle parts. At right, you can the proper restraining method for making any intravenous injections.

the choke rope, the vein become enlarged and rigid because of back pressure. If the choke is sufficiently tight, the vein stands out and can be easily seen and felt in thin-necked animals.

As a further check in identifying the vein, tap it with your fingers in front of the choke rope. Pulsations that can be seen or felt with the fingers in front of the point being tapped will confirm the fact that the vein is properly distended. It is impossible to put the needle into the vein unless it is distended. Experienced livestock producers are able to raise the vein simply by using hand pressure, but the use of a choke rope is more certain.

Properly placing the needle into the vein involves several distinct steps:

1 Insert the needle through the hide.Insert the needle into the vein. This may require two or three attempts before the vein is entered. The vein has a tendency to roll away from the point of the needle, especially if the needle is not sharp.

2 The vein can be steadied with the thumb and

finger of one hand. With the other hand, the needle point is placed directly over the vein, slanting it so its direction is along the length of the vein, either toward the head or toward the heart. Properly positioned, a quick thrust of the needle will be followed by a spurt of blood through the needle—indicating the vein has been entered.

3 Once in the vein, the needle should be inserted along the length of the vein all the way to the hub, exercising caution to make sure the needle does not penetrate the opposite side of the vein. A continuous steady flow of blood through the needle indicates the needle is still in the vein. If blood does not flow continuously, the needle is not in the vein (or clogged) and another attempt must be made. If difficulty is encountered, it may be advisable to use the vein on the other side of the neck.

4 While the needle is being placed in proper position in the vein, have a helper get the medication ready so the injection can be started without delay once the vein has been entered.

5 Remove the rubber stopper from the bottle of intravenous solution, connect the intravenous tube to the neck of the bottle, invert the bottle and allow some solution to run through the tube to eliminate all air bubbles.

6 When making the injection, make sure the needle is in proper position as indicated by a continuous flow of blood. Then release the choke rope by a quick pull on the free end. This is essential as medication cannot flow into the vein while the vein is blocked.

7 Immediately connect the intravenous tube to the needle and raise the bottle. The solution will flow into the vein by gravity. The rate of flow can be controlled by pinching the tube between the thumb and forefinger or by raising and lowering the bottle.

8 Bubbles entering the bottle through the air tube or valve indicate the rate at which the medication is flowing. If the flow should stop, this means the needle has slipped out of the vein (or is clogged) and the procedure will have to be repeated.

9 Watch for swelling under the skin near the needle which indicates the medication is not going into the vein. Should this occur, it is best to try using the vein on the opposite side of the neck. Sudden movement of the animal, especially twisting of the neck or raising or lowering the head, sometimes cause the needle to slip out of the vein. To prevent this, tape the needle hub to the skin of the neck to hold the needle in position. Whenever there is any doubt as to the position of the needle, this should be checked by pinching off the intravenous tube to stop flow, disconnect the tube from the needle and re-apply pressure to the vein. Free flow of blood through the needle indicates it is in proper position and the injection can then be continued.

10 When the injection is complete, remove the needle with a straight pull. Apply pressure over the area of injection for a few seconds to control any bleeding through the needle puncture. Use cotton soaked in alcohol or another suitable antiseptic.

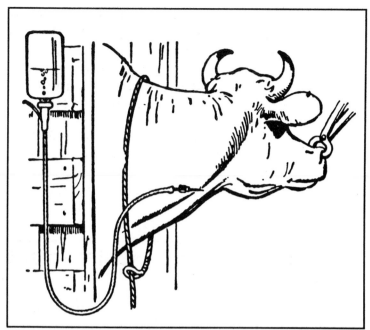

PROPER POSITIONING. This shows the correct position for the bottle, tube and needle in making an intravenous injection. Note that the choke rope is loosened to allow for the proper flow of blood in the vein. This is very essential.

Injection Precautions

To reduce the likelihood of shock, intravenous solutions should be warmed to approximately the animal's body temperature before injection.

Rapid injection may occasionally produce shock. Administer medicines slowly. The rate of injection may be controlled by raising or lowering the bottle or by pinching the tube. The animal should be observed at all times during the injection so as not to give the solution too fast.

This may be determined by watching the respiration of the animal and feeling or listening to the heart beat. If either the heart beat and/or respiration rate increase markedly, the rate of injection should be immediately stopped. Do this by pinching the tube until the animal recovers to its previous respiration or heat beat rate. Then the injection can be resumed at a slower rate.

If symptoms of shock are seen or the animal shows any signs of distress, administration can be interrupted by pinching the intravenous tube. If symptoms persist, the injection should be terminated entirely.

Making An Intramuscular Injection

An intramuscular injection is made through the skin and subcutaneous tissue, directly into the muscle. Absorption is very rapid in this case.

Needed Equipment

- A 25 or 50-cc veterinary syringe.

- Hypodermic needles, 16 gauge, 3/4 to 1 in. long.

- Scissors or clippers.

- 70% rubbing alcohol compound or other equally effective antiseptic for disinfecting the skin and bottle stopper.

- The medication to be given.

Preparing The Equipment

Clean and disinfect the needles and syringe by boiling in water for 20 minutes.

Areas Of Injection

An intramuscular injection is made directly into the muscle tissue or meat. All intramuscular injections should be made ahead of the shoulder in the neck region.

Not more than 25-cc of medicine should be injected in any one spot in large animals such as cattle. Where the dosage to be given is large, as much as 500-cc can be injected into cattle by distributing the dosage in 25-cc amounts.

Preparing The Animal

Restrain the animal by the best means available. A stanchion or chute is ideal for large animals. Clip the hair from the area where the injection is to be given. Swab the clipped areas vigorously with alcohol or other equally effective antiseptic.

Making The Injection

By following these ideas, you can be sure that these types of injections are made properly:

☛ Fill the syringe with the medication to be given, using a separate needle for filling. Disinfect the rubber stopper before inserting the needle into the bottle.

☛ Insert a previously disinfected needle deeply into the muscle tissue with a quick thrust. Observe the hub of the needle for a moment. If blood begins to flow out of the needle, it is probably in a blood vessel and the needle should be withdrawn and reinserted in a different direction. Attach syringe to the needle and inject the medication slowly.

☛ After the medication has been injected, remove the needle still attached to the syringe and massage the area with cotton soaked in alcohol to spread the medication through the muscle tissue.

☛ These procedures should be repeated in each injection area until the full recommended dose of medication has been given.

Making A Subcutaneous Injection

A subcutaneous injection is made into the tissue beneath the skin.

Be sure to read the directions for making an intramuscular injection. The equipment needed, its preparation and preparation of the animal are the same as for an intramuscular injection.

A subcutaneous injection is an injection made beneath the skin, usually between the skin and the muscle tissue. Recommended areas of injection are where the skin is loose, particularly on the sides of the neck and behind the shoulder.

To make the injection, pinch up a fold of skin between the thumb and fingers. Insert the needle under the fold in a direction approximately parallel to the surface of the body. When the needle is inserted in this manner, the medication will be delivered underneath the skin between the skin and the muscles. Observe the same precautions regarding clipping and disinfecting the skin as outlined under intramuscular injections.

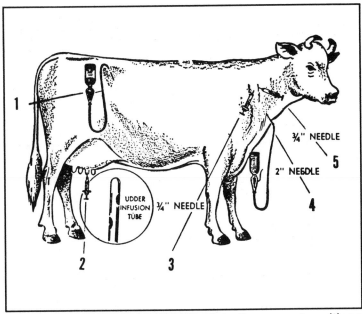

CATTLE INJECTION GUIDES. Note the correct positions for making injections in cattle. For more detailed instructions follow the step-by-step procedures which are outlined in full detail in this chapter.

1. Intraperitoneal injection—right side only with 2 in. needle. (Not recommended except by your own veterinarian).

2. Udder infusion—for mastitis treatment.

3. Subcutaneous injection—under the skin. Examples would be blackleg bacterin whole culture (alum treated), brucella abortus vaccine, anti-hemorrhagic-septicemia serum and chauvei-septicus-pasteurella (triple bacterin).

4. Intravenous Injection—jugular view. This would include injections of sterile glucose solution, anti-hemorrhagic-septicemi serum, anti-corynebacterium-pasteurella serum, sodium cacodylate solution, triple-sulfa solution, sodium iodide solution and thio-nitro solution.

5. Intramuscular injection—deep into the muscle. Examples would include mixed bacterins, hemorrhagic-septicemia bacterin, corynebacterium-pasteurella bacterin (whole culture), blackleg bacterin (whole culture), camphoil, sterile glucose solution, sodium cacodylate solution, globestrol and penicillin.

Other Methods Of Administering Drugs

Several other methods of administering drugs to cattle are as follows:

Inhalation

(Inhale). Volatile drugs are used mainly for their local action on the respiratory tract.

Rectal

By the rectum. This method is used when oral administration is inadvisable or impossible due to paralysis of the throat, etc. Absorption of medication is slower.

Topical

This includes local application of medicines to external surfaces of the body. Absorption by this method is extremely slow and the effects of the drug are limited to the treated area.

Oral

Some drugs are given through the mouth and are absorbed in the stomach and intestines. Absorption is more rapid when drugs are given in a solution into an empty stomach; much slower when administered in powder, pill or ball form or on a full stomach.

Chapter 17

A Quick, Easy Way To Throw Your Cattle

THERE ARE many occasions when mature cattle must be thrown and held in a prone position to facilitate handling. These occasions include surgical operations, the treatment and dressing of wounds, trimming overgrown hooves and many other important management practices.

While throwing a heavy cow or bull may appear to be a formidable job, it is surprisingly easy to do providing a few simple rules are followed. All the equipment you need is a rope and halter.

Steps To Take To Throw An Animal

First, the animal should be driven into a yard, paddock or large box stall and tied by a halter. The leadrope from the halter is then held by an assistant or it can be secured temporarily with a couple of turns around a post or fence rail. Under no circumstances, should it be tied in any way which will not allow you to release it quickly. You may need to slack it off very quickly when the animal goes down and you should plan accordingly before going ahead.

Next, take a 30 to 40 ft. length of strong rope (approximately 1/2 in. or more in diameter) and tie one end around the back of the animal's neck or fore-shoulders using a bowline or some other type

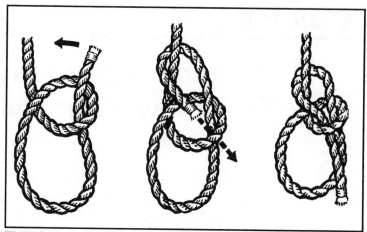

TYING THE PROPER KNOT. To make a non-slip bowline knot, follow the steps outlined in this illustration. You will find many uses around the farm for this very common knot.

of easy-to-tie, non-slip knot.

This loop should serve as a loose-fitting collar and the lower part can be loose enough to fall down across the animal's brisket. If the animal has horns, the loop may be placed around them instead of around the animal's shoulders. The non-slip knot for the shoulder loop serves to prevent possible choking of the animal when the actual pulling starts.

Follow These Instructions

With the loop attached around the shoulders and secured with a non-slip knot, carry the rope back over the withers and put a half-hitch around the animal's body just behind the forelegs. You make the half-hitch by dropping the end of the rope to the ground on one side of the animal, passing it under the belly, coming back up the other side and then going under the rope, over the shoulders.

Take up the slack and continue to carry the rope back over the animal. Make another half-hitch encircling the body just in front of the hip bones.

In the case of a cow, the lower part of the half-hitch should be placed in front of the udder to avoid bruising the milk producing tissues. If the animal is a bull, pad the bottom part of the loop with cloth or a grain sack to avoid possible injury to the penis when the rope is tightened.

The long end of the rope is then carried back behind the animal and slightly to the side on which you want to throw it.

Easy Does It

Take up the slack in the rope and you are now ready to throw the animal. Check again to see that it is tied or haltered so pulling the rope will not simply pull the animal backward. Then start a strong, steady pull (avoid jerks) on the rope which should

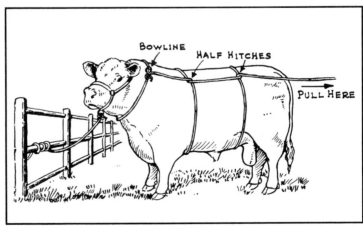

HITCHING UP THE ROPE. Here's how the rope should be placed and appear when you are ready to throw the animal.

cause the animal to go down gently without any type of struggle.

A cow will usually remain motionless as long as a steady pull is maintained on the rope. For long operations, however, it is a good plan to take precautions and tie the legs together with an extra rope.

This simple casting device is strikingly effective. Even a large and powerful bull will go down slowly and smoothly in a manner which never fails to amaze the inexperienced onlooker.

The method is presumably effective because the rope exerts pressure on vital nerve centers in the animal's body.

Chapter 18

Properly Trimming The Feet Of Your Cattle

IT'S VERY EASY to keep the feet of your cattle neatly trimmed.

Proper trimming of hooves prevents sore feet, quarter cracks and costly lameness. This is especially true with cattle, but also applies to sheep and swine.

Trim 'Em Early

Cows should normally have their feet trimmed at

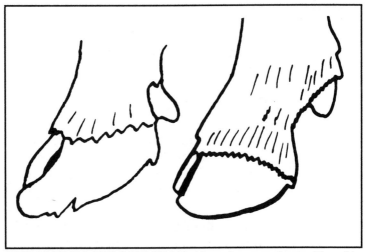

RIGHT WAY, WRONG WAY. Here is a neglected hoof in need of trimming (left) and a properly trimmed hoof (right).

8 or 9 months of age and again at regular intervals thereafter as needed.

The outside of the hoof should be trimmed back with hoof nippers. A sharp, wide chisel or rasp should be used on the bottom of the foot to make it flat and even. This trimming process shortens the hooves and levels the bottom of the foot so the animal walks and stands straight on its feet and legs.

Legs And Feet Are Important

Poor care of an animal's feet develops improper leg growth among other things. Many cattleman state that "cows with poor legs and feet never develop into old, useful animals." It is also known that dairy and beef cattle with neglected feet do not graze well and consequently drop in milk and/or meat production.

Slick Ways To Trim Feet

There are many known ways to trim the feet of cattle. Long toes are sometimes cut off with a saw or chisel. This does some good, but it doesn't correct the improper position of the foot.

This can only be done by properly paring the bottom surface of the claws as well as the forward growth of the "toes." Usually the heaviest paring is necessary on the toe end of the foot.

Gentle beef and dairy animals will usually allow their feet to be trimmed while in a standing position. This is best done by using a pair of long-handled trimmers which are especially made for this particular purpose.

When done in a standing position, the animal should stand on bare ground or flooring so bedding and other materials do not interfere with the cutting of the hooves.

There is no sure way to tell how far back the edges of the hooves can be cut, since there are wide individual differences in hoof structure. However, hooves resemble human fingernails and can too easily be cut back into the "quick" to cause pain, bleeding and an opening for possible infection.

It is thus best to remove only a small segment of the hoof edge at a time to obtain the desired shape. If bleeding starts, it is a certain sign that trimming has been carried too far and should be stopped at once.

Trimming The Soles

Trimming the soles of an animal's feet will require raising one foot at a time unless the animal has been thrown. With the foot raised off the ground, either the long-handled trimmers, hoof pinchers or hoof rasp can be used for removing part of the soles.

Nervous animals which have a tendency to kick will require raising the feet before trimming of any kind can be done properly and safely.

One method of raising and trimming the hind hoof with the help of two men is to wrap a burlap sack around a metal rod. With a man on either side of the animal and with the rod in front of the hock joint, lift the leg upward and slightly backward.

Another method to raise the hind foot and avoid being kicked is to place two half hitches above the hock around the hind leg of the foot to be trimmed, throw the other end over a beam or through a pulley and pull the leg up.

Many other methods of trimming are also used. One is a box- like table made of wood planks about 10 to 12 in. high. The hoof is then placed on the table and in this position can be readily pared down to the desired shape with a knife or chisel.

There are also a variety of stocks suitable for confining an animal to trim its feet.

Trimming Tools To Use

These are the tools that you should have on hand when preparing to trim an animal's feet:

- A T-shaped handle welded onto the shank of a

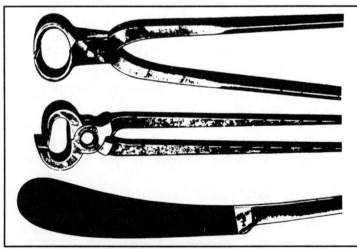

THREE KEY TOOLS. From the top of this illustration down: Hoof nippers, hoof parer and hoof knife for trimming.

wide chisel makes a very satisfactory tool in paring off the bottom of the hoof. Gentle persuasion and skill are necessary for this operation.

- In addition to this homemade tool, a hoof rasp for smoothing, a hoof pick to clean cracks and crevices, wire brush for cleaning the surface and hoof knife for paring are handy tools.

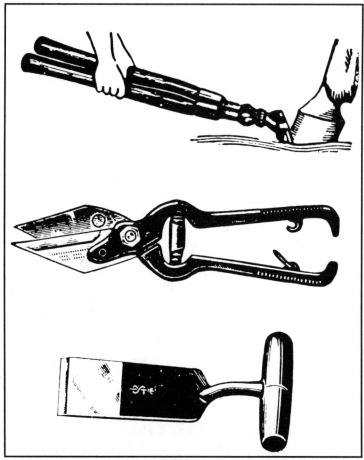

TOOLING UP FOR TRIMMING. Use these common tools for proper hoof care. At top, a popular, long-handled tool for trimming cattle feet in a standing position. At center, a sheep foot rot shear. At bottom, the shortened chisel for hoof trimming which is described in full detail in this article.

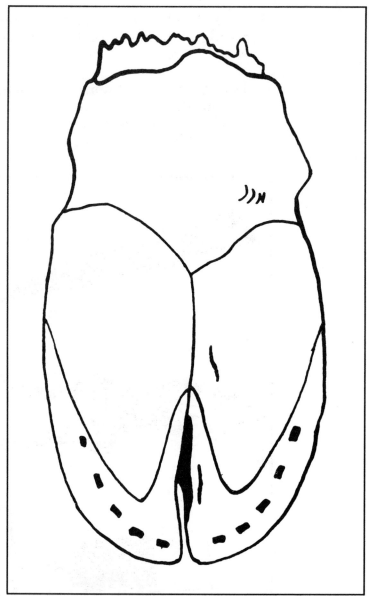

HOW TO TRIM A HOOF. Use this illustration as a guide for proper trimming. However, simply remove only a small part of the hoof at a time to avoid cutting into the "quick". The dotted line near the edge of the hoof indicates the amount which is usually trimmed off. Above the dotted line is the sensitive area or "quick." Cutting into this area often causes pain, bleeding and may even result in an infection.

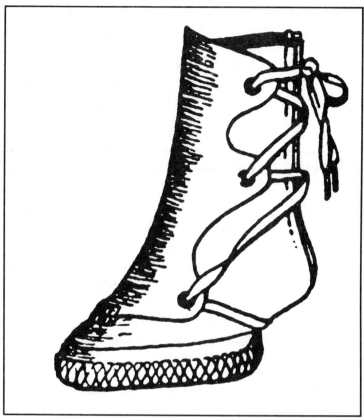

GIVING HOOF ROT THE BOOT! For hoof rot, the cow boot shown here assists in bringing infection under control. Without a cow boot, it is nearly impossible to keep the hoof clean and dry and give medication a good chance to work.

To use the cow boot, clean the hoof thoroughly and apply a good antiseptic. Sulfa powder is an effective treatment. Spread dry bicarbonate of soda between the toes and add a teaspoon in the bottom of the boot to keep the boot dry.

Softening The Hoof

To reduce the physical effort involved in cutting off

a long hardened hoof on a cow, stand her in clean mud several hours a day for a short period of time. Then, cut off the extended part if the hoof and treat it sparingly with a hoof oil (applying too much oil tends to make the hoof waterproof and prevents the proper absorption of moisture which is needed to keep it in normal condition).

Applying Hoof Oil

One oz. of turpentine or 1 oz. of coal oil mixed in enough neats-foot oil to make a pint serves as a good hoof oil. Tallow, wool fat, lard and pine oil may also be used. A mixture of wool fat and tar is also excellent to soften brittle hooves.

Remember that proper care of the hoof is the start of better and healthier livestock in your herd or flock.

Chapter 19

Dehorning Your Cattle And Calves

CATTLE WITH HORNS definitely need more space, particularly in confined building situations. They are inclined to fight and keep other cattle away from feed. They are also more dangerous to handle and can injure other animals.

Dehorning Method Depends On Age

Very young calves can be dehorned by applying caustic or commercial dehorning paste to the horn buttons. Slightly older calves with horns or horn buttons not over 1/2 to 3/4 in. long can be dehorned easily with heated dehorners. Older animals must have their horns removed with mechanical devices, hand saws or electrical saws.

The sooner that dehorning can be done, the less your animals will suffer. Young animals are much easier to handle and also have fewer after effects.

Restraint Is Necessary

A combined branding and dehorning chute with one movable slide (known as a "squeeze") is widely used in western range country to hold cattle for dehorning. On farms where branding is not a common practice, chutes with stationary sides are

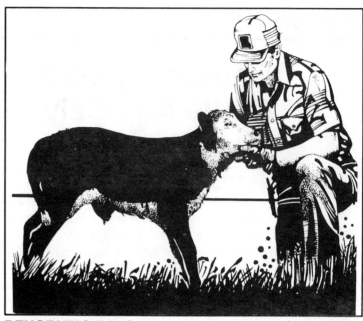

DEHORNING PAYS. While it may cost you $1 to $3 per animal for dehorning, the expected return from using this management practice will range from $5 to $15 per head.

often used. In all cases, large animals must be tied or held securely.

Disbudding, Dehorning Calves

If treatment is done before the calf is 10 days old, caustic soda or potash can be used to dehorn your calves. First clip the hair around the base of the small, undeveloped horns or buttons and apply vaseline to the area surrounding the buttons to prevent the caustic from touching the skin. Caustic applied directly to unprotected skin burns it, irritating the calf and causing the animal to rub the spot and weaken the chemical.

To apply the caustic, wrap one end of a caustic stick

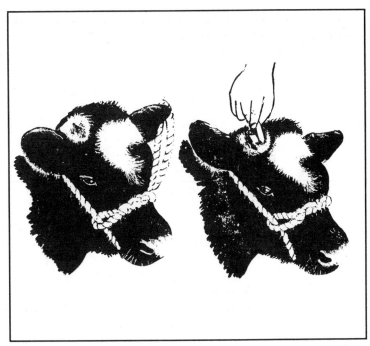

EARLY DEHORNING. If calves are dehorned before reaching 10 days of age, caustic soda or potash can be used. However, take precautions to keep the caustic off of the calf's hair as it will seriously burn any unprotected skin.

in paper or cotton and moisten either the exposed end of the stick or the horn button. Moisten lightly because too much water may cause the caustic to flow out of the horn button site. Rub the horn button and an area around it about as big as the size of a nickel with the caustic. The degree of destruction of the horn growth area depends on the number of applications, pressure used, area covered and the amount of moisture. Calves dehorned with caustic should be protected from rain for a few days following treatment.

If dehorning paste is used to dehorn calves, cover the horn button with a dime's thickness of paste applied with a stick. No preliminary clipping is necessary.

Dehorning Older Calves

Calves past the button stage are best dehorned with heated irons, metal spoons, gouges, tube dehorners or Barnes-type dehorners. The type of instrument best suited to a particular operation depends largely on horn size. The horn should always be removed with a ring of skin to prevent further horn growth.

Spoon and tube gouges work best on calves under 60 days of age. Different sizes of dehorning tubes can be purchased. To use, select the size that fits over the base of the horn and includes about 1/8 in. of skin around the horn. Place the cutting edge straight down over the horn. Push down and twist until the skin around the horn has been cut

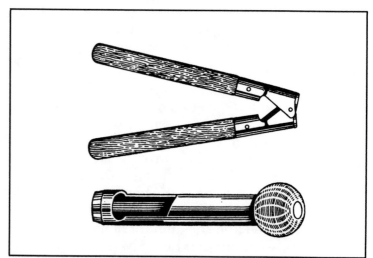

DEHORNING CHOICES. Barnes type dehorner, top, is especially adapted for dehorning calves. Available in several sizes, a larger unit can be used for dehorning animals up to 1 year old. The tube dehorner, bottom, slips over the horn to first cut a ring around a small-sized horn before removing it. These tube dehorners come in different sizes.

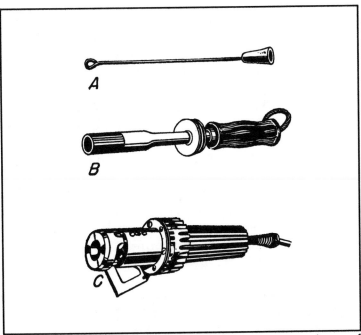

HEATED DEHORNERS. Item A is a common type of dehorner which is available in different sizes and is used immediately after heating in a fire or portable heater. B and C are other types of electric dehorners that are available.

through 1/8 to 3/8 in. deep. Older calves will require the deeper cut. Then turn the spoon down to a 45-degree angle and lift the horn button out.

Barnes-type dehorners can be used more easily on larger calf horns than other instruments. They are also used to dehorn yearlings or older cattle. To use a Barnes-type dehorner, simply close the handles and fit the knives over the horn. Make certain the knives are correctly positioned to remove a 1/2 in. collar of skin along with the horn. Pull the handles apart quickly, thus closing the knives and removing the horn.

The hot-iron method of dehorning is widely used in western range country. Since the development of electrically heated irons, this technique is becoming more widely used in farm-size beef and dairy herds. It is commonly used to dehorn calves up to 4 or 5 months of age.

The hot-iron method of dehorning is reasonably rapid and practically bloodless. Irons other than the electric type are usually sold in sets. Select the size that fits the horn to be removed.

Heat the copper-capped head of the iron to a cherry-red heat, then slip it over the horn or horn base for about 2 minutes until a copper-colored ring has been burned around the base of the horn. The horn or button will slough off within 4 to 6 weeks.

Dehorning Older Cattle

The dehorning clipper is the most efficient instrument for dehorning older cattle. To use it, place the opened blades over the horn and quickly close the long handles. Make the cut deep enough to remove a 1/2 in. wide collar of hair and skin along with the horn. The deep cut exposes the larger blood vessels in the soft tissue and gives them an opportunity to contract, thereby decreasing the amount or post-operative bleeding.

When larger animals are dehorned, bleeding can be minimized by using forceps to pick up the main artery on the ventral or under side of the cut. Pull the artery until it breaks. The end of the broken artery will retract—going back into the softer tissues—and bleeding stops. If you can find the artery, there will probably be little bleeding. The most important thing about pulling an artery is to do it with clean, sterile instruments.

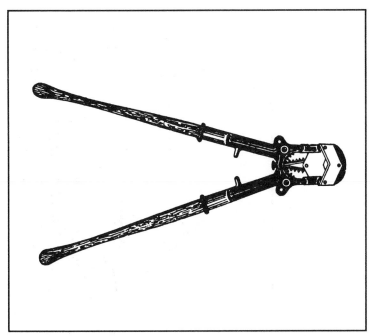

LARGE HORNS. This dehorning clipper is used for removing the horns from older cattle. Various sizes are available.

Dehorning saws can be used for trimming the ends from horns or for removing the entire horn. Their use is necessary when the horn base is too large for clippers or when abnormal horn growth prevents using clippers. When saws are used for a complete job of dehorning, cut deep enough to remove a ring of skin and to prevent later growth of abnormal, unsightly horns.

Electric dehorning saws can lessen your time considerably, save labor and minimize discomfort to the animal. Electric saws are more expensive than other types of dehorning equipment and their disinfection is more of a problem since the entire machine cannot be submerged. The blades must be swabbed with disinfectant.

When dehorning saws are used, local anesthetics

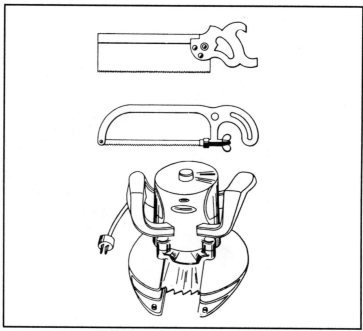

DEHORNING SAWS. With dehorning saws, livestock producers prefer the stiff blade, miter-type saw at the top. The electric dehorner, bottom, is another valuable instrument.

are usually administered to eliminate any animal pain. Cows in lactation and in advanced pregnancy can then be dehorned without seriously affecting milk production or jeopardizing pregnancies. In most states, you can buy local anesthetics where you buy your veterinary supplies. Administer with a syringe according to instructions.

Controlling Bleeding

Bleeding after dehorning usually isn't serious in calves, but it is best to find ways to control it when older animals are dehorned.

The best procedure calls for locating the ends of

bleeding arteries and pulling them out so they break below the cut surface. A pair of surgical hemostats or small-nosed pliers can be used for pulling out these arteries.

Another method consists of tying a piece of twine completely around the poll or head well below the cutting line of the horns. When drawn tightly, it will press on the arteries entering the base of the horns to cut off the flow of blood.

On some cows, you may be able to tie the twine around the individual horn well down the side of the head. If desired, a heavy rubber band or cross section of an old inner tube can be used instead of twine. Either the twine or rubber band should be watched and removed within several hours or less to prevent gangrene around the poll region. This is important.

Dust, flour, cobwebs and similar materials should never be used for the control of bleeding after dehorning. They don't do much good and they can start an infection in the opened sinuses of the head.

Feeding moldy sweet clover hay or silage increases bleeding, too. So avoid all surgery if this is the case.

Disinfecting Instruments

Instruments that are used for dehorning, especially those which come in contact with blood, should be disinfected with the utmost care. This should be done before and after each operation. It is especially important in areas where anaplasmosis is prevalent or suspected.

Wash used instruments in cold water to remove

blood. Then soak them in a compound solution of cresol or saponified cresol (also called cresylic disinfectant). Mix the solution by adding 4 oz. of cresol to 1 gal. of water. Put the dehorning instruments directly into the solution and use them immediately after removal. Change the diluted solution frequently so its strength can be adequately maintained.

Treating Horn Wounds

If dehorning is done in cool weather when there are no flies, wound treatment is unnecessary. Take precautions to see that dirt, manure or other filth does not contaminate the wound. Certain infections are soil or filth borne. Provide clean, well-bedded stalls or clean pastures for dehorned animals.

If dehorning is done in warm weather, it usually is necessary to apply a fly repellent such as pine tar to the wound.

In the southern states, severe screw worm infestations are not uncommon. Do not dehorn during screw worm season. If necessary, just remove the tips of sharp horns. Apply a commercial smear or spray to control screw worm. Apply a light coating to uninfested wounds caused by dehorning. To treat infested wounds, work this material in well and apply a coating completely around the wound. Give special attention to any deep pockets made by worms. Repeat this treatment twice a week until the wounds are healed.

There are some precautions to take in the use of screw worm smear or spray materials. For these reasons all directions which accompany the product should be read and carefully followed.

Chapter 20

Castrating Your Calves

ALL MALE CALVES which will not be used for breeding purposes on the farm or ranch should be castrated. Castrating is essential to the production of a high quality carcass. It also helps prevent inbreeding and the breeding of females in the herd by undesirable males.

Like the task of dehorning, castrating should be performed in cool weather to prevent serious infections. Between the ages of 1 and 3 months is considered the ideal time to do it, although many cattlemen prefer to castrate when calves are only 1 or 2 weeks of age.

Generally speaking, the younger the calf, the less inconvenience it suffers and the quicker it completely recovers. It is best to castrate calves from 1 to 2 months of age, since it causes less pain and is more humane. The calf can also be implanted at this time.

Castration is best done from a position where you stand directly behind the animal. Your vision is better and the danger to you from the animal kicking is much less.

It is done easiest on standing animals after they have been confined in a chute or stanchions and restrained by the tail. Of course, if the animal to be castrated is rather large, it must be thrown as explained in another part of this manual.

How To Hold Calves

Restraining calves by the tail is a very effective means for holding them for castration, for removing extra teats on heifers or for other health work that may encourage kicking.

It is done by raising the tail in the air with one hand so it can be grasped near the base of the tail with the other hand. Forcing the tail toward the animal's head has a restraining effect because the feet can't be raised without hurting the animal's back. You will need one person to restrain the animal and one to handle the procedures.

Before starting the operation, all instruments should be thoroughly cleaned and sterilized by boiling and scrubbing them in a solution of alcohol. If alcohol isn't available, scrubbing in good hot soapy water will do the job.

There are two common methods of castrating calves with a cutting instrument. They are equally effective. So far as we know, there is no more danger of infection from using either method than the other.

Lateral Or Side Incision Method

Follow these steps for successfully using this method of castration:

☞ After the calf is adequately restrained, grasp the scrotum with the thumb and forefinger of the left hand so as to stretch the skin tight over the right side of the right testicle.

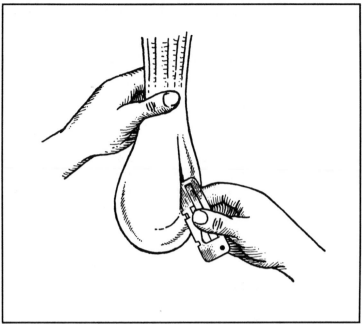

LATERAL OR SIDE INCISION. A slit is cut with the knife down the right side of the scrotum, starting a few inches above the top of the testicle and then ending just below it.

☛ With your knife in your right hand, cut a slit down the right side of the scrotum, starting a few inches above the top of the testicle and ending a little below it. This incision must be deep enough to cut through all layers of skin and tissue and expose the testicle. This incision may end up being deep enough to cut into the testicle itself.

☛ Grasp the exposed testicle with one hand and with the other hand, strip the spermatic cord attached to the testicle of all its loose surrounding tissue so the cord is exposed well up to the top of the scrotum.

☛ Pull the testicle down with the left hand, exerting a slight pull (about 2 lbs. pressure) and separate the testicle from all of its supporting tendons. While still holding the testicle with the left hand, cut these tendons (not the spermatic cord) close to their lower attachments on the testicle.

☛ Be sure the remaining spermatic cord is stripped of all surrounding membranes. Draw the cord down as far out as possible and sever or separate it by scraping with the blade edge of the knife. Less bleeding results if the cord is cut in two by scraping. Make this cut high—up near the animal's body to remove as much spermatic cord as possible.

☛ Repeat these procedures to remove the remaining testicle.

☛ Take care to avoid infection. Clean the area where the incisions are made and apply disinfectant or antiseptic powder.

If this task must be performed during the fly season, apply a fly repellent to the skin surface around the incision. Do not be in such a hurry as to avoid this step. Castration should be performed in cool weather when there aren't flies if at all possible.

End Incision Method

This is the more commonly used method for castrating calves. You perform it by following these all-important steps:

☛ Grasp the bottom of the scrotum with the left hand and squeeze it to force the testicles upward and out of the way.

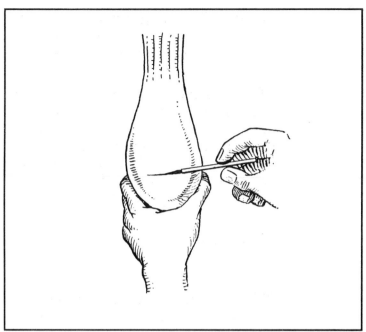

END INCISION. With this more commonly used method, make a cross-wise cut around the sac one-third of the way up on the scrotum. Remove this bottom third of the sac.

☛ About one-third of the way up on the scrotum, start cutting cross-wise or around the scrotal sac. Completely encircle the scrotum and remove the bottom third. This leaves the testicles dangling uninjured and encased in a sac called the "tunic." Nick or cut the "tunic" with the knife and a testicle will be exposed.

☛ Grasp the testicle with one hand. With the other hand, strip the spermatic cord from its surrounding tissue. Expose the cord well up near the top of the scrotum.

☛ Next, pull the testicle down with the left hand, exerting a slight pull (about 2 lbs. pressure) and separate the testicle from the supporting tendons.

While still holding the testicle with the left hand, cut these tendons (not the spermatic cord) close to their lower attachments on the testicle.

☛ Check the remaining spermatic cord to see if it is stripped of all surrounding membranes, then draw the cord down as far as possible and sever or separate it by scraping with the edge of the knife. Less bleeding results if the cord is severed or cut in two by scraping. Make this cut as high up near the animal's body as possible.

☛ Repeat these steps to remove the remaining testicle.

☛ Take the needed precautions to avoid any infection. Clean the skin where incisions are made and apply disinfectant or antiseptic powder.

If this operation must be performed during fly season, apply a fly repellent to the skin surface around the incision. Do not skip this step! Castration should be performed in cool weather when there aren't flies, if possible.

Caring For Animals After Castrating

After reasonable care is taken to avoid infection, a castrated animal should be left alone in a stanchion or pen. A pen that is clean is better than a stanchion because the animal is more at ease. However, it is not a good idea to place the animal in a pen with uncastrated calves because they may become excited and run around—causing further strain on the castrated calf.

While the calf may not eat or drink for several

hours after you finish, this is not unusual after this kind of serious operation.

The castrated animal usually requires no special care if it is placed in a clean, quiet place. But it pays to keep a careful eye on the animal from day-to-day to check for the possibility of any infection or serious bleeding. Infections or unusual bleeding are rare. If they do occur, they should be treated immediately by a veterinarian.

Calf Castrating Equipment

The type and condition of the castrating knife you use is extremely important. A dull knife makes castrating difficult. Your knife should be sharp to do a fast, sanitary and safe job.

The most satisfactory castration knife for calves

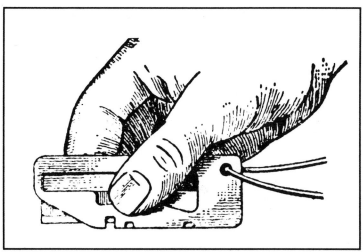

NEAT CASTRATING KNIFE. For castrating calves and smaller animals, it is hard to beat the type of knife shown here. Featuring an easily-replaed razor blade, it slides in and out of this holder to limit and control the depth of cut.

and smaller animals, holds a sharp, but easily replaced, low cost razor blade. A protected blade slides in and out of the holder to limit the depth of cut. It gives you assurance that your incisions are under control at all times. As an extra convenience, this type of knife can be attached to a cord that goes around your neck to free both hands when not actually using the knife.

Still another good castrating instrument is the scalpel. The old fashioned castrating knife is also acceptable—providing you can keep it sharp.

Good disinfecting powders and solutions suitable for use on castration wounds are also available. One recommended low cost powder is a combination of sulfa powders and urea. Sprayed or puffed onto the wound, it helps avoid infection and facilitates healing.

This particular section of this book covers only the castration of calves by cutting into the scrotum and removing the testicles. Other methods of castration with the emasculatome, emasculator and rubber band elastrator for each particular species of farm animal are covered in separate sections of this book.

Chapter 21

Using Your Beef Cow Record Sheets

IF YOU REALLY want your beef cows to produce at the most effective rate, there is no substitute for keeping good records. There's probably no one management practice that will earn you a bigger return than analyzing a good set of records.

Over the years, it has been proven many times that the selection of beef animals and herd replacements by sight is not a satisfactory method for a cattle producer to use. While an animal's type can generally be seen with the eye, productive ability, which is the real value of any beef cow, is spread out over a long period of time and is much more difficult for a cattleman to judge.

Well-kept, up-to-date beef records enable you to know exactly what your animals have done—not what you think they may have done in your herd. Since you cannot always remember everything you do with your beef animals, writing it all down in a set of beef records is very essential to success.

The logical time to start keeping record cards on your beef cows is just prior to calving time. If you get your beef records set up prior to calving time, you can record valuable calving information as it occurs.

To help you keep the right kind of records, the publishers of this book have put together beef cow records which you can easily use. Details on purchasing the beef cow record sheets shown in this chapter are found in the front of this book.

Steps In Using Your Record Cards

Assign one beef record card to each cow. Write down her identification number along with other useful information for which spaces are provided at the top of the card.

Mark each cow to permanently identify her. Ear tattoos, neck chains, brands and ear tags are common identification methods which are used by successful cattleman.(See chapter 22 for full details on using various methods of animal identification).

While ear tattoos are probably the best identification method, owners of purebred or small herds may prefer neck chains. For cattle running on the range, branding along the side of the animal will make identification much easier.

Breeding Record

List the date the cow was bred, the bull used and the date when the cow or heifer is due.

Once she calves, record calving ease, the date and sex of the calf in the provided spaces on the card. There is also room on this record form to later show what happened to the calf.

Health Record

List all health management information in this portion of the card. This should include all infor-

FRONT OF BEEF CARD. The front of this beef cow record card contains plenty of room for listing the breeding history and production record of both the animal and its offspring.

mation regarding treatment dates, symptoms, diagnosis, treatment and results so you can look back at this in-depth information later on when trying to decide what to do health-wise for a particular animal.

Production Record

Space is provided on the back side of the card to show the identification number or mark of the calf, birth weight, weaning weight, grade and adjusted weaning weight. (You will find more on determining adjusted weaning weights at the end of this chapter).

This part of the card serves as the "real meat" of your beef record system since it will tell you which cows are producing the calves that earn you the most money.

Try to "work" each of your calves within the first

Beef Calf		Record Sheet		Cow ID _____				

Production Record

Year	Calf Identification	Birth Weight	Actual Date	Weaning Pounds	Weight Grade	Adjusted Weaning Wt	Remarks

Veterinary Record

Calf Number	Date Born	Date Castrated	Vaccination, Additive or Implant Record		
			Date	Material Used	Purpose

BACK OF BEEF CARD. The back of this beef cow record card provides room for keeping a history of both veterinary and health dates, symptoms and treatments for the animal.

few days after birth. Get the birth weight, sex, dam number and sire number written down if it is known. Mark the calf either temporarily or permanently. Some cattlemen like to use temporary tags attached to the calf's ear with a hog ring to avoid the time involved in rechecking a calf which has already been worked.

Veterinary Record

This part of the card allows you to keep valuable and useful information about all health work done with the calf. List dates of castration, implants, any additives used, vaccinations, other health treatments and a record of diseases which may affect the beef cow or its calf.

These detailed records will later prove to be a valuable guide for both you and your veterinarian.

Better Records, Better Beef Herd

The overall success of your beef management program will depend a great deal on the kind of records you keep. By keeping detailed breeding, health, production and veterinary records such as those shown in this chapter, you will be able to do a better job of managing your beef herd.

The result will be a herd that improves in quality, enjoys higher production rates and one that will bring you a very profitable return.

A Word About Weights

Birth weight is an important indication of how a calf will produce later in life. Research shows birth weights are closely related to weaning weight, final feedlot weight and gains while on feed. Calves which are heavier at birth tend to grow faster and gain more efficiently in order to produce beef at the lowest possible cost.

A bathroom scale can be used to take birth weights in the field. With the scale on level ground, weigh both yourself and the calf. Deduct your weight and you will have the net weight of the calf.

These scales can fit into an oversized saddle bag quite easily. Your other saddle bag can hold a tattoo marker, temporary marker tags, hog rings, ringer and any other equipment which is needed in the field.

Grading Your Calves

Calves should be graded for you by one, two or three unbiased graders. Just ahead of weighing at weaning time, list the grades on the record card. The more graders you use, the more accurate should be the grade arrived at for each calf. Authorities agree that the most accurate grading is done before, not after, weighing.

Weaning Weights

As already stated, calves should be weighed again at weaning time. This is best done with a portable scale mounted on a two-wheel trailer. Grading and weighing takes only about 2 minutes per animal with this equipment.

Adjusting Weaning Weights

Since it is impractical to weigh all calves at exactly the same age, it is usually necessary to adjust weaning weights so that a number of calves can be compared. To permit grading all calves on an equal basis, adjust all weights to "steer equivalent".

The best method is to weigh all your calves at 6 to 8 months of age. While opinions differ as to just what age is best for this adjustment base, judging from available facts, any time within the 2-month range will do.

The adjustment weight is computed by taking the calf's weaning weight and dividing this by its actual age in days. This gives the weight per day of age. Multiply this figure by 240 (8 months) to get the adjusted 8 month weaning weight.

As an example, let's use a calf weaned at 250 days of age with a weaning weight of 500 lbs.

The 500 lbs. divided by 250 days equals 2 lbs. weight per day of age.

The 2 lbs. times 240 days equals 480 lbs. adjusted weight.

This weight must be further adjusted to allow for the sex of the calf and the age of its dam. Both of these factors must be accounted for in order to get the "steer equivalent" for each calf.

The sex of calves is adjusted for by adding 25 lbs. to the adjusted weaning weights of heifers and by subtracting 25 lbs. from the adjusted weaning weights of bull calves.

Adjustment for age of the dam is also very important in your beef herd because experimental data from a number of universities shows there is a marked increase in weight of the calf as a cow approaches 6 to 8 years of age. After a cow reaches

Additions To Weaning Weights To Correct For Age Of Dam

Age	A	B	C
2 years	45 lbs.	36 lbs.	70 lbs.
3	40	24	50
4	20	16	30
5	5	8	15
6	0	0	10
7 and 8	0	0	0

8 years of age, the birth weight of her calves will begin to fall off.

Adjustment factors for age of dam from universities in three states are shown in this chart. It makes little difference which scale you use so long as you use it for all calves.

Now, adding to the example used previously, we will assume the calf was a bull and came from a dam that was 4 years old. We subtract 25 lbs. from the 480 lbs. adjustment weight (adjustment for bull calf) and, using the scale for state A, add 20 lbs. for a dam that is 4 years old. Thus: 480 lbs. adjustment weight minus 25 lbs. plus 20 lbs. equals a final adjusted weaning weight ("steer equivalent") of 475 lbs.

This weight now serves as a simple numerical index to effectively compare one calf in your herd with another. It should be recorded on your Beef Cow Production, Breeding, and Health Record Cards in the space provided under the column headed "Adjusted Weaning Weight".

The higher this number, the better the calf, providing he has good physical characteristics visible to the eye.

Chapter 22

Marking, Branding Your Beef Cattle

THE POPULARITY OF branding and marking as a means of properly identifying cattle has been growing since the earliest days of cattle raising in the United States. Both still are widely practiced despite many changes taking place in methods used for handling cattle.

Branding and marking are not frequently used where farms are small. A limited number of cattle can be identified from natural markings or with neck chain markers.

However, where cattle are raised in large pastures or out on the open range, branding is usually considered necessary. Range cattle often are earmarked as an additional means of identification.

Branding Is Really A Trademark

A cattleman firmly believes his brand is his trademark. Most successful ranchers take pride in their brands and guard them closely. In all cattle-raising states, particularly in the range area, the law deals severely with people found guilty of changing or tampering with brands or marks.

Letters, numerals or other characters comprising the brand should be of a design that is easily made. Intricate characters lead to confusion in reading brands as well as difficulty in branding. They should be avoided.

In some western states, the law requires branding of all livestock which are turned out on the range. Nearly all western states require that records be kept of brands on all slaughtered animals. Cattle brands used within a state ordinarily are registered and recorded by a department of the state government.

Cattle that change ownership are often rebranded. When this occurs, old brands are blotted or crossed out.

Cattle are branded officially in the eradication of bovine tuberculosis and brucellosis (Bang's disease). Eradication projects are conducted cooperatively by the federal government and the states. Animals that react to the tuberculin test are branded on the left jaw with a letter T; those that show a positive reaction to the test for brucellosis are branded on the left jaw with a letter B.

Age At Branding

Cattlemen usually brand calves before they are weaned. This is because the probability of a calf going astray is much greater after it is weaned.

Early branding lessens the possibility of such losses. When disputes arise as to ownership of a calf, it is customary to concede ownership to the owner of the cow that claims the calf. This is particularly true where open range is used or where mixing with other cattle is probable.

Methods Of Branding

Methods of branding include: applying a hot iron, using a cold iron dipped in a commercial branding fluid or freeze branding using a frozen iron. Each method, if properly carried out, leaves a permanent mark.

Cattle to be branded are thrown or squeezed in a chute. Throwing of animals has given way somewhat to various methods of chute branding because branding can be done more easily in a chute. If chute branding is done, the location of the brand on the animal should be one which can be easily reached through the bars of the chute.

It is difficult to build a chute or squeeze that will securely hold both small calves and older cattle. Conventional-type chutes are satisfactory for branding animals over 1 year of age.

Improved tilting tables are satisfactory for calves. Several types of tilting tables for calves are on the market. All operate on a movable or turntable base. The calf is secured to the "cradle" and the unit is given a 90-degree turn. It falls into position with the calf held securely on its side.

Chute-branding older cattle is better than throwing them, but care must be taken in closing the squeeze chute. It is easy to crush the hip of an animal being confined in a powerful squeeze. The leverage of a squeeze should not be so great that the operator fails to perceive the degree of pressure he applies.

Types Of Branding Irons

The two general types of branding irons being used today by cattle producers are "running" irons and "stamping" irons. Running irons are simple hooks. Both types of irons are used for hot branding, but a stamping iron is much better for liquid branding.

There is little defense for using extremely large characters in a brand. A character 4 in. high is large enough for identification purposes, especially if the brand is applied when the animal is young. Characters with narrow angles should be avoided if a stamping iron is used, as letter divisions are often not refined enough to prevent blotching when the iron is heated.

Open letters such as O, C, D, P and Q can be made distinctly with a stamping iron. Letters such as A, M, N, W and X usually can be made with a running iron by making the required number of applications to complete the letter.

Branding irons should be made with notches where the bars join. The faces should be be leveled and smooth. The rod of bar iron or steel from which the characters are made should be large enough to hold enough heat, yet small enough to make a neat line. Material between 1/4 and 1/2 in. in diameter is commonly used. Material which is 3.8 in. in diameter is a popular, desirable size for hot-iron branding.

Hot irons need handles at least 2 1/2 ft. long to permit easy handling by the livestock producer. Stamping irons for liquid branding have concave faces and shorter handles.

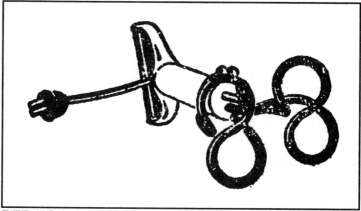

RED HOT. An electric branding iron heats fast and maintains proper branding heat during use. With generators and converters now available for vehicles, electric branding irons are even being used successfully out on the range.

Elastic branding irons are stamp irons made from nichrome steel. The amount of heat they deliver can be varied and regulated. They often are used for electric dehorning saws and electrically heated dehorning irons.

Applying The Brand

Keep all of your branding irons free from rust and out of the weather when they are not being used.

Hot-Iron Branding

Wood is the best fuel for a branding-iron fire. Before applying a hot iron, make sure it is hot, but not too hot. When properly heated, the iron should be ash gray.

Deep burning is cruel and unnecessary. If the hide surface if merely scorched, the brand usually peels and remains distinct. Slipping an iron usually results in a poor imprint on the animal.

Wet or damp animals cannot be branded successfully. The brand will scald or leave a blotch, a bad sore or no imprint at all.

Liquid Branding

When using this method, dip the iron in about 1/8 in. of branding fluid which has been stirred thoroughly. Apply the brand to a surface that has short, dry hair.

It is difficult to control the depth of liquid brands. If they are applied too lightly, they will soon disappear.

It is also difficult to keep these brands from becom-

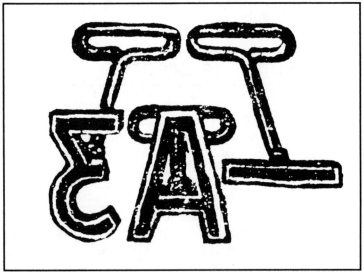

FROSTY COOL. Cold branding irons are made to brand cattle without requiring the use of a hot iron. A chemical liquid compound produces a lasting brand on livestock, providing the iron is carefully used according to directions.

ing distorted. Water on the raw branded surface will cause the burn to spread. Distortion also occurs if the animal licks it or switches it with his tail before the fluid dries. For these reasons, this form of branding isn't very popular.

Freeze Branding

The advantages of freeze branding over a hot iron are that it is relatively painless, is permanent and leaves no costly scars. Scarred hides cost the beef industry millions of dollars every year.

With freeze branding, animals stay on feed and infections from open wounds and screw worms are not problems.

The current method is to chill copper branding irons, (although steel or bronze have also been used) in a dry ice-alcohol bath to -158 degrees F. The iron is placed against the animal's clipped hide for 30 seconds. A welt appears for a short period of time and then all hair is shed from the brand area, usually within 22 days.

Freeze branding destroys the pigment in the hair and skin, leaving a white mark on the skin and new hair. White animals can be marked by leaving the iron on longer. This permanently destroys the hair and removes skin pigment within the branded area.

Drawbacks include the length of time it takes to cool the iron versus heating it, higher cost and not knowing whether the brand has "taken" until hair regrowth actually takes place.

Branding Considerations

The following are branding recommendations from the Montana Livestock Commission:

☛ Choose a good brand, one that is distinctive and readily recognized. The recorder of marks and brands in your state can aid you in selecting a brand which has the desired qualities within limits imposed by brands already on record.

☛ Have your choice of a brand recorded. Unrecorded brands afford little or no protection and result in much confusion with consequent loss and waste.

☛ Apply the brand properly. It should be on the position recorded, of sufficient size to be readily seen and should be clearly and cleanly burned in with a hot iron having faces at least 3/8 in. wide. Letters, figures or characters should be 4 in. long.

☛ Provide a proper bill of sale when selling any brand of animal. Protect yourself and others by insisting that the buyer take a completely and properly filled out bill of sale.

☛ Demand a proper bill of sale on all purchased animals. Be particular as to brands and the legal requirements of the bill of sale. By doing so you will save yourself much trouble, annoyance and expense in future transactions.

☛ When offering cattle for sale which carry brands other than your own, be prepared to prove your ownership.

☛ To avoid delays, give your local inspector as much advance notice as possible when regulating brand inspections.

Marking The Ears

The practice of marking cattle by cutting the ears is almost as widespread as branding and usually is done at branding time.

It is not uncommon for cattlemen to perform all operations—castration, health shots, branding and marking—at the same time. Earmarks are rather secondary to branding, although they are recorded in the brand records and are protected by law.

Either or both ears may bear a mark. Marking is done so cattle can be identified from the front or rear. It often is difficult to get a side view of wild cattle running in a pasture or on the range.

A sharp knife should be used in marking cattle as the cartilage of the ear usually is tough and clean cuts should be made. Some of the more common marks are described here.

Crop

Fold the ear length-wise and make the cut at right angles to the folded edge.

Overslope

Make an incision a fraction of an inch from the point, toward the head, where the upper surface of the ear turns up. Cut down approximately 1/2 in.,

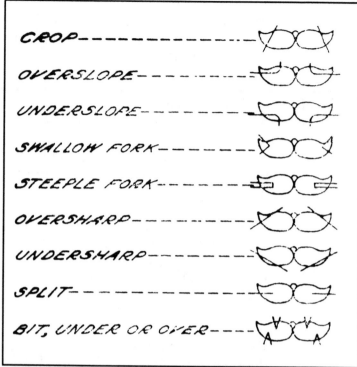

CROP

OVERSLOPE

UNDERSLOPE

SWALLOW FORK

STEEPLE FORK

OVERSHARP

UNDERSHARP

SPLIT

BIT, UNDER OR OVER

CREATIVE MARKS. These illustrations show the common earmarks that are used for identifying cattle. All of these earmarks are explained in more detail in this chapter.

in a rounding manner and then cut outward parallel to a line that would halve the ear lengthwise. A little upward slope given to the last cut gives a graceful curve.

Underslope

The underslope cut is on the underpart of the ear. The first cut is made in an upward manner. The second cut is practically the same as that made in an overslope.

Swallow Fork

Fold the ear lengthwise. From a point 3/4 in. or 1 in. from the tip, depending on the size of the ear, cut toward the outer edges in such a direction or manner that a triangular section with 1/2 or 3/4 in. base will be removed.

Steeple Fork

Fold the ear lengthwise. Make the first cut at right angles to the seam and the second cut parallel to the seam. Remove a rectangular section of the ear.

Oversharp

This cut is begun at the same point as for an overslope, but brought downward and in a straight line to the median line at the tip of the ear.

Undersharp

Cut in a straight line between the same points as in making an underslope.

Split

The knife blade is inserted and drawn to the outer edge of the ear.

Bit, Under Or Over

Fold the ear crosswise at the point where the bit is to be made. Remove a triangular section as in making a swallow fork.

Tattoo Identification

Tattooing the ears is a method of marking cattle which is especially adapted for use with purebred herds.

It is considered a more permanent method of identification than cutting the ears. Tattooing is done with a special instrument that places characters, letters or numerals in and under the skin of the ear by means of a series of needle-like points dipped in a special indelible ink before application. The op-

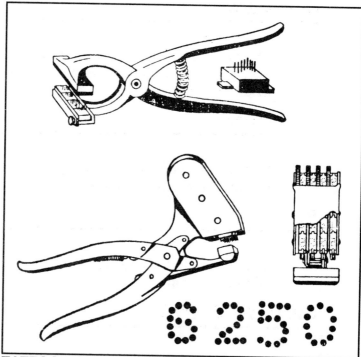

TATTOOING CHOICES. Here are the various types of tattooing instruments which are used by cattle producers. Above, is an inexpensive simple type with interchangeable numbers and letters. Below, a rotary type tattoo suitable for large herds and in situations where speed is important.

eration is simple and does not leave any open wound. It is advisable to apply additional ink to the ear after the perforations have been made to insure the permanence of the identification. Tattooing instruments can be obtained from most dealers who handle stockmen's supplies.

Eartagging Works

Like tattooing, eartagging is another method of identification that is used largely with purebred herds.

Metal tags or buttons are clamped into the ear with special clamps. The tag or button carries the necessary identification numbers or letters.

Neck Chains

In some instances, owners of purebred cattle prefer not to make permanent identifications with earmarks, eartags or tattoo marks in the ears. Instead, they use neck chains that carry special identification numbers.

Chains for this purpose may be purchased from many supply houses.

Hip Brands

Still another option for marking cattle is the use of hip brands bearing identification numbers. This type of marking is often more desirable than neck chains where cattle run on the range.

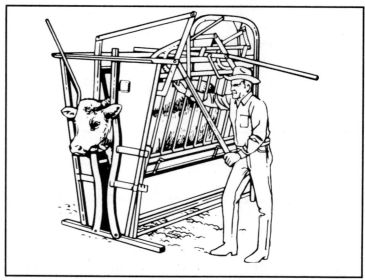

LOTS OF CHUTE OPTIONS. Squeeze chutes, which have a removable side, are ideal for use when branding or treating cattle. Animals can be held more securely in these types of chutes than in chutes featuring stationary sides.

Working Chutes

Chutes made with one movable side—called squeezes—hold animals snugly and safely under pressure and can be used when cattle are branded, castrated or vaccinated. They are better that stationary-sided chutes because animals can be held more securely.

Several commercially-made squeeze chutes are available. Ease of operation and construction costs should be considered in deciding whether to buy or build a chute.

A chute with stationary sides is easier to construct and is satisfactory where small numbers of cattle are handled.

Chapter 23

Diseases, Management Of Your Beef Cow Herd

HERE IS A quick rundown on a number of animal diseases that can certainly create problems for you in your beed herd:

Brucellosis

Age Affected: All ages of beef cattle.

Prevention: Test and remove all reactors. Repeat three times. Vaccinate all heifers and calves at 3-6 months.

Treatment: None.

Tuberculosis

Age Affected: Usually occurs in older animals.

Prevention: Periodic testing. Remove reactors.

Treatment: None.

Leptospirosis

Age Affected: All ages of beef cattle.

Prevention: Vaccination for five serotypes.

Treatment: Dehydrostreptomycin.

Drug Withholding Period: 30 days.

Calf Scours

Age Affected: 1 to 4 weeks of age.

Prevention: Vaccinate your cows 3 weeks prior to calving. Give 2 qts. colostrum to calf at birth. Offer Diaproof orally when scour symptoms appear.

Treatment: Electrolytes, antibiotics and sulfas.

Drug Withholding Period: Ranges from 5 days to 30 days.

Coccidiosis

Age Affected: Usually under 1 year of age.

Prevention: Prevent stress, particularly at weaning time when coccidiosis is apt to be present.

Treatment: Feed 22.7 mg of Decox per 100 lbs for 28 days.

Drug Withholding Period: None.

Vibriosis

Age Affected: Animals of breeding age.

Prevention: Vaccination prior to breeding.

Treatment: None.

Bovine Virus Diarrhea

Age Affected: Young beef animals.

Prevention: Vaccination with a killed virus.

Treatment: Supportive treatment.

Infectious Bovine Rhinotracheitis

Age Affected: Primarily young animals.

Prevention: Vaccination.

Treatment: Supportive treatment.

Bovine Syncytial Virus

Age Affected: Primarily occurs in animals up to 1 year of age.

Prevention: Vaccination.

Treatment: Supportive treatment.

Bacterial Pneumonia

Age Affected: This occurs primarily in animals up to a year of age.

Prevention: Eliminate stress. Vaccination prior to exposure.

Treatment: Chlortetracycline 350 mg per head per day or Sulfamethazine fed at a rate of 350 mg per head per day.

Drug Withholding Period: 8 days for chlortetracycline. 48 hours for Sulfamethazine.

Rabies

Age Affected: All ages of beef cattle.

Prevention: Vaccinate of all farm cats and dogs.

Treatment: None

Lump Jaw

Age Affected: All ages of cattle.

Prevention: This is caused by sharp objects penetrating an animal's body tissue.

Treatment: Streptomycin I.M.

Drug Withholding Period: 30 days.

Clostridial group (7)

This vaccination program includes treatment for Blackleg Malignant edema, Red Water, Enterotoxemia and Sordelli.

Age Affected: Primarily occurs in animals up to 1 year of age.

Prevention: Vaccination.

Treatment: Penicillin I.M.

Drug Withholding Period: 5 days.

Pinkeye

Age Affected: Young animals are most susceptible.

Prevention: Control of flies. Vaccination.

Treatment: Inject antibiotics over eye. Patch over eye. Sew eyelids closed.

Drug Withholding Period: 5 days.

Listeriosis

Age Affected: All ages of cattle.

Prevention: No vaccine available.

Treatment: Antibiotics.

Anaplasmosis

Age Affected: All ages.

Prevention: It can be spread from infected animals to susceptible animals by knife, needles or insects. Chlortetracycline at a rate of 350 mg per head per day can help prevent the disease.

Treatment: Chlortetracycline at a rate of 500 mg per head per day.

Drug Withholding Period: 5 days.

Bloat

Age Affected: All ages. It primarily affects animals grazing legumes or cattle on full feed.

Prevention: Use Polyoxyaline or Bloat Blox.

Treatment: For the release of gas from the rumen, use Polyoxyaline.

Foot Rot

Age Affected: All ages of cattle.

Prevention: Zinc methionine at a rate of 4 grams per head per day.

Treatment: Sulfas or antibiotics.

Drug Withholding Time: 5 to 10 days.

"Water Belly"

This common health problem with beef cattle is also known as urinary calculi.

Age Affected: This is primarily a problem in young steers.

Prevention: Add 1% to 2% salt to your rations. Or feed ammonium chloride at a rate of 0.75 to 1.25 oz per head per day.

Treatment: Surgery.

Internal Parasites

Age Affected: All ages of cattle.

Prevention: Carry out a strategic deworming program. Worm adult animals in the spring and fall. Treat calves when they weigh 200 lbs.

Treatment: There are several excellent dewormers on the market available in many different forms—pastes, injectables, pellets and minerals. Select the dewormer that has the broadest spectrum (gets all species of worms) and kills the immature worms. Cost should also be considered as some dewormers cause twice as much as others.

Drug Withholding Time: Ranges from 5 to 8 days. Check the product label.

Lice

Age Affected: All ages of beef cattle.

Prevention: Use a spray, pour-on or dip product.

Treatment: Use your choice of Co-Ral, Ciodrin, Malathion or Warbex.

Drug Withholding Period: Follow label instructions.

Chapter 24

Treating External Parasites In Beef Cattle

USE THIS INFORMATION as a guide in determining how best to prevent unnecessary problems and to properly treat all of your beef animals for external parasites.

Lice

Prevention: Use a backrubber or spray your animals. However, spraying is probably the best method of louse control in beef cattle. In addition to killing lice with spraying, enough insecticide will remain in the hair and coat of the animal to later kill lice which hatch from eggs several days after application. While use of backrubbers will suppress louse populations, they will not effectively eradicate lice.

Treatment: There are a wide variety of spray materials and backrubber chemicals available for treatment. Talk with your veterinarian about the product which will be best to use under your particular circumstances.

Drug Withdrawal Period: Check labels carefully as some spray materials have specific drug withdrawal requirements.

Mange

Prevention: Spray or dip. Mange is a reportable disease to state veterinary health authorities and your animals will be quarantined on the premises.

Treatment: Most states have control and eradication programs. Check with a local veterinarian as to required chemical usage.

Flies

Prevention: Fly control with pastured cattle is difficult. It can be accomplished with use of low-level feed additives, backrubbers, dust bags, oilers or sprays.

Treatment: You can use a wide variety of dust bags, sprays, pour-ons, spot treatments, backrubbers and ear tags and tape strips for fly control.

Drug Withholding Period: Check labels carefully as some products have 7 to 35 day withdrawal requirements prior to slaughter.

Insecticide Ear Tags, Tapes

Prevention: Insecticide ear tags and tapes provide a convenient, effective method of fly control on pastured cattle. However, horn flies have developed resistance to these products in some parts of the country.

Producers who have used pyrethroid ear tags or

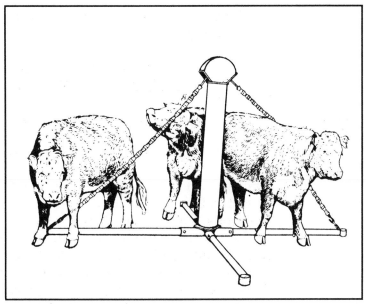

MANY OPTIONS. Cattle producers have a wide range of methods and products to choose from when it comes to controlling external parasite problems in their beef herds.

tapes in the past may want to consider using alternative control measures. These alternatives include the use of organophosphate insecticides applied as sprays, dust bags, backrubbers, pour-ons or feed additives.

Treatment: There are several different types of fly tags now on the market. The following guidelines are recommended for their effective use:

- With most tags, fly control is not very effective after 6 months from the the date of application. To avoid applying tags too early, wait until a few flies appear. The chances of developing some type of resistance is also greater at the end of the fly season.

- Rotate to a different type of tag each season. Be sure to place a tag in each ear of every animal.

- Remove all tags 6 months from the time of application.

- Also be sure to use other methods of fly control along with tag usage.

Grubs

Prevention: Treat your beef cattle for grubs from Aug. 1 to Dec. 1 to avoid unnecessary chemical side reactions. Learn the life cycle of the two species of grubs to fully understand the reasoning behind this recommended insecticide treatment period. Grubby animals are not only expensive to the producer, but are not good for the image of the beef industry. Grub control will also provide needed louse control for your cattle.

Treatment: A number of spray and pour-on insecticides can be used to control grubs. Check with your veterinarian for his suggestion as to which product he feels you should be using.

Drug Withdrawal Period: There are various drug withdrawal requirements for some of these materials. Some insecticides cannot be used on calves under 3 months of age and some products should not be used with Brahman cattle. The drug withdrawal period may also depend on the particular formulation of the product you are using. Check the label carefully.

Chapter 25

Preventing, Treating Coccidiosis In Cattle

COCCIDIOSIS FREQUENTLY hits all groups of cattle, but sometimes most severely affects those animals in the feedlot. However, the most frequent victims are often young calves.

Coccidial parasites are always present where cattle are housed. These protozoa are commonly found in the digestive tract of the cattle. Carrier animals can contaminate pens, paddocks and pastures. Calves under stress, especially at weaning time, are likely candidates for coccidiosis infections.

Outbreaks of coccidiosis depend upon two factors:

• The number of sporulated or infective oocysts (infective stage of coccidia).

• The susceptibility of animals to the infection.

Many Causes Of Coccidiosis

Ample moisture, warm or mild temperatures and contamination of feed, water and bedding with manure containing the oocysts (the infective form of coccidiosis) help in spreading the disease. Overcrowding and filthy conditions are usually seen in coccidiosis outbreaks. Any procedure that reduces moisture, temperature or contamination will help control coccidiosis.

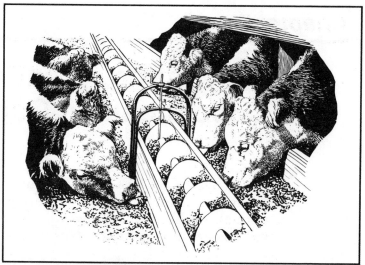

RECOGNIZING THE PROBLEM. One of the biggest treatment problems with coccidiosis is the failure to recognize when the inital attack takes place. This is very critical so all treatment can be timed properly with clinical symptoms.

The mere fact that the infective form of the coccidia is ingested by your animals does not mean an outbreak of the disease will occur. The animals themselves must also be in a susceptible stage.

Fatigue from shipping, sudden changes in weather, sudden changes in feed, such as going from roughage to concentrates or the addition of a new feed ingredient which may change the conditions of the digestive tract, predisposes animals to coccidiosis.

The greatest period of susceptibility occurs during the first few weeks of confinement. During this time the oocyst intake may be continuous and may reach a troublesome buildup range at 3 to 6 weeks. If all animals are housed in the same lot and exposed to the same conditions, an explosive outbreak may occur. Coccidiosis infections are usually self-limiting and subside to a low grade infection in 10 to 14 days with lasting immunity to follow.

It is thought that high concentrate rations are actually more conducive to coccidiosis than most roughage rations. This is because of their texture, moisture content and resulting impact on the animal's digestive tract.

Prevention Ideas

The prevention of coccidiosis is easier to discuss than to actually implement. Rapid fattening of animals in crowded pens produces ideal situations for initial attacks. Calves started out slowly in the feedlot will develop a resistance to coccidia without showing severe symptoms. While these calves or feeders may actually have mild infections, they may not show severe symptoms since they are not on full feed with intestinal upsets. Feeding coarse, dry roughage with small amounts of concentrates and taking 6 to 8 weeks to reach full feed usually prevents coccidiosis.

The use of coccidiostats (Decoquinate given at 10 mg per kg) for 5 days is recommended as a preventative for recently weaned calves, new animals in the feedlot or when young animals are congregated together. Coccidiostats are effective as preventives, but not as treatments.

If coccidiosis strikes, the following precautions should be immediately followed:

1 Be sure it is coccidiosis and not an enteritis of some other cause.

2 Isolate infected animals. They are rapidly shedding the organisms which can quickly create a total feedlot problem.

3 Mass treatment is recommended. Use of drugs in water or feed will inhibit the multiplication of coccidia before the lining of the intestine is attacked by the parasites.

Time Treatment With Initial Attack

For successful treatment, time your treatment with the initial attack. Treatment may be repeated in 10 to 14 days if the timing of the first treatment has been correct.

The biggest problem to date with treatment has been a failure to recognize the initial attack so treatment can be timed with clinical symptoms. Cattle have been known to lose 50 to 75 lbs. from coccidial infections. In some instances, death has occurred.

The nervous form of coccidiosis has been found in some feedlots where a few infected animals show serious central nervous disturbances. It is felt this is due to toxins liberated by the coccidia, but this idea has not been definitely proven.

Chapter 26

Beef Cattle Herd Health Program

This recommended month-by-month herd health management program, with suggested health, nutrition and management practices, was developed for use by any beef producer who is following a spring calving program.

January

Health

Be on the lookout for scabies. Watch for abortions. Treat for lice.

Nutrition

For each 10 degree drop in winter temperature below 15 degrees, add 1.5 lbs. of total digestible nutrients (TDN) to the ration.

Management

Provide a minimum of 5 gal. of ice-free water per day for each of the cows, heifers, bulls, steers and calves in your herd.

February

Health

Watch for foot rot. Vaccinate cows with Clostridium perfringens to prevent some type of scours in calves when born. Check on using a vaccine that prevents virus-produced and E. coli-type scours in calves. These vaccines must be given prior to calving. They have proven to be of value.

Nutrition

Increase energy and protein needs by 2 lb. of total digestible nutrients and 0.2 lb. of crude protein.

Management

Check pregnancy exam records to determine calving dates. Prepare calving quarters. Have heat lamps on hand for early calving. Plan ahead so that calving does not occur in mud and filth.

March

Health

Provide a clean, dry calving facility. Have heat lamps on hand. Know how to feed weak calves, if necessary, with a stomach tube. A calf must have colostrum within 6 hours of birth. Some serums are available that can replace colostrum. Have them on hand just in case for the calf that can't nurse.

Nutrition

Provide a minimum of 9 lbs. total digestible nutrients before calving and up to 16 lb. after calving. Feed and manage first-calf heifers and old cows separately from the rest of the herd.

Management

Record birth dates. Separate non-pregnant cows and identify calves.

April

Health

Deworm all cows. Provide grass tetany prevention with magnesium oxide (0.5 oz per cow per day) mixed in a mineral mixture. Deworm all cows before turning them on pasture.

Nutrition

Plan your pasture program. Feed dry hay before turning cows out on succulent pasture.

Management

Identify difficult calving cows on your records. Castrate and implant 1 to 2 month old calves. Purchase sires for this year's breeding program. Make final selection of heifer replacements. Watch for cows in heat. Record essential herd information.

May

Health

Fertility check bulls. Vaccinate open cows for vibriosis, IBR, BVD, Leptospirosis (five serotypes) and Haemaphilies somnus BRSV 30 days prior to breeding. Vaccinate all of your calves and young stock for pinkeye.

Nutrition

Watch carefully for grass tetany problems. Feed 0.5 oz of magnesium oxide per day per head. Watch for bloat. Use bloat preventative blocks or mixes.

Management

Start breeding heifers, one cycle ahead of your cows. Set up fly control measures. Use tags or tapes. Set up other types of fly control such as dustbags and sprays.

June

Health

Get ready to use artificial insemination. With natural breeding, use one bull (fertile) for 25 cows. Check on the use of estrus synchronization products. Cows must be cycling properly in order to settle. Estrus synchronization will work if management factors are used as recommended.

Nutrition

Provide creep rations. Good pasture should carry
your cows, but pasture supplementation may be
necessary in some cases.

Management

Creep feed depending on pasture availability and
grain prices. Check prices of commercial creep
feeds and formulas for home-mixed creep feeds.

July

Health

Vaccinate all calves over 3 months of age for pinkeye, Clostridial group (Blackleg, etc.), Pasteurella
and Haemophilus BRSV. Vaccinate heifer replacements with Strain 19 at 2 to 6 months of age.

Nutrition

Check pastures for poisonous weeds, insecticides
and fertilizer buckets and bags. Supplement pastures if needed.

Management

Consider weaning calves now if your pasture is
short. Reinforce fly control measures. Check cows
for evidence of their return to estrus for rebreeding.
Deworm and reimplant all calves.

August

Health

Check on pinkeye problems and treat any affected problem animals at once with antibiotics.

Nutrition

Plan your winter feed supply. Check each cow's condition and supplement if necessary.

Management

Remove bulls. Reimplant calves with the same type of implant that was used previously. Deworm cows and calves.

September

Health

Watch for grass tetany. Check for foot rot and cancer eye. Check on fly control measures.

Nutrition

Watch supplementary crops for frost damage. Include magnesium oxide in feed.

Management

Plan your calf program carefully. Early weaning of calves at 5 to 6 months of age is recommended.

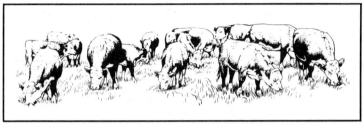

FOLLOW THE CALENDAR. By managing your beef herd with specific health, nutrition and management practices each month, you should earn a very excellent profit return.

October

Health

Pregnancy check all cows. Vaccinate calves while you are pregnancy checking cows. Vaccinate for IBR-PI3 killed BVD, Clostridial group, Haemophilus and BRSV. Deworm both cows and calves and treat for external parasites.

Nutrition

Provide supplementary forage as needed.

Management

Cull your cows and back tag all cows going to slaughter.

November

Health

Process calves, wean and sell all feeder calves.

Nutrition

Supplement roughage if necessary. Feed protein and concentrate.

Management

Select replacement heifers.

December

Health

Check cows for abortion, heat periods.

Nutrition

Check feed supplies and winter rations for your cows. A cow should gain 100 lbs. during her gestation period.

Management

Feed first-calf heifers separately from older cows. Dispose of bulls which will not to be used during the next breeding season.

Chapter 27

Cost Effectiveness Of Using Recommended Beef Cattle Practices

Following the 10 critical beef management recommendations outlined in this chapter will aid you in obtaining a 95% calf crop while producing a 600 lb. calf at weaning time. Remember that you are producing pounds of beef and not just raising a certain number cattle each year. An 80% calf crop should be considered as your breakeven number.

Check out the proven economic returns you can earn from using these key management practices in your beef operation:

Deworming

- *Cost Per Animal:* $1 to $2.50 for a calf and $2 to $5 for a cow.

- *Expected Return Per Animal:* $10 to $30 per head for calves and $10 to $40 for cows. Figure an average return of $10 per calf and $25 per cow.

60 Day Pregnancy

- *Cost Per Animal:* You can earn an extra 50 cents per cow per day for each day 60 days after calving when a cow is pregnant.

- *Expected Return Per Animal:* $30 to $60 for each cow/calf pair. Anticipate an average return of $45 for your investment in on-time breeding.

Fertility Testing

- *Cost Per Animal:* Your costs should run $20 to $30 for each bull tested and $2 for each cow that undergoes a fertility examination.

- *Expected Return Per Animal:* Each fertility checked cow should return $10 to $20 per head. Figure on an average return of $15 per cow.

Castrating Bull Calves

- *Cost Per Animal:* It will cost you $1 to $3 per head to do.

- *Expected Return Per Animal:* You should be able to earn an extra return of $10 to $20 per calf. Expect an average return from improved gains of $15 per steer calf.

Dehorning

- ***Cost Per Animal:*** Your costs will run $1 to $3 per head.

- ***Expected Return Per Animal:*** You should be able to earn an extra $5 to $15 per head, with an average return of $10 per head from dehorning.

Implanting

- ***Cost Per Animal:*** Your costs will run $1 to $2 per head.

- ***Expected Return Per Animal:*** Look for a $12 to $25 per head return from implanting, with an average return of $18.50 per head.

Vaccination

- ***Cost Per Animal:*** It should cost you $2 to $3 to provide the necessary vaccinations for your cows. Vaccinations for a calf will run $3 to $6 per head.

- ***Expected Return Per Animal:*** You should earn a return of $5 to $15 per head with a cow, with an average return of $25 per head. Expect a $10 to $20 per head return with calves, with an average $15 per head return.

Pregnancy Checking

- ***Cost Per Animal:*** These examinations normally cost $2 to $3 per cow.

- ***Expected Return Per Animal:*** This practice should return $20 to $30 per cow, earning you an average return of $25 per head.

Crossbreeding, Tested Bulls

- ***Cost Per Animal:*** Figure on investing an additional $10 per head for crossbreeding and use of production tested bulls.

- ***Expected Return Per Animal:*** Your returns from using these practices will run $20 to $30 per head, with an average return of $25.

Records, Identification

- ***Cost Per Animal:*** Figure on spending $1 to $2 per head for good animal identification and record keeping.

- ***Expected Return Per Animal:*** You should be able to earn an extra $5 to $10 per head from properly identifying animals and keeping good records. Your average extra return should be around $7.50 per head.

Chapter 28

Using The Proper Implanting Techniques

THE USE OF growth-stimulating drugs as pellets implanted subcutaneously in the ear of beef animals has become a common management practice for many cattle feeders.

According to reports from nutritionists, veterinarians and feedyard managers, unsatisfactory responses to an implanted drug often result from improper implanting technique. The use of the correct technique in administration of any implant will mean a 10% to 15% advantage to the animal in the form of better weight gain and increased feed efficiency.

Absorption of the implanted drug depends upon several factors:

- Shape and size of the pellet.

- The carrier that is used.

- Hardness of the pellet.

Optimum pellet shape, size, carriers and hardness have been selected by implant manufacturers through detailed studies measuring actual amounts of absorption.

Common Implanting Errors

Your techniques in using the implanting gun or other implanting device has just as great or perhaps a greater effect upon absorption of the drug than physical characteristics of the implant pellet. Common implanting errors include:

1 Gouging the cartilage of the ear.

2 Intradermal rather than subcutaneous implantation.

3 Severing one of the veins of the ear, causing hemorrhage.

These errors may be avoided by careful use of the implant gun. If any of these errors are committed, absorption of the drug by your cattle will probably not be effective.

When the cartilage in the ear is gouged, pellets may be crushed. If crushing occurs, absorption of the drug will probably be too rapid. A rapid rate of absorption may cause development of side effects or, at the least, will reduce growth response. Implants deposited in gouged cartilage may be covered with scar tissue and "walled off." This will result in virtually no absorption of the drug.

Intradermal implanting occurs when the needle is inserted between several layers of skin. Poor absorption of the drug will result and no response to the drug will be observed.

Hemorrhage due to cutting or piercing one of the

veins in the ear may result in a too rapid absorption of the drug. When the pellets are immersed in blood, they soften and disintegrate. As the blood is reabsorbed, the drug will be absorbed at a rate which is more rapid than desired. In such cases, growth response will be considerably less than expected.

Implanting Techniques

Properly administered implant pellets will be absorbed over a period of time and the drug will provide the desired growth stimulation. Proper implanting is relatively simple. However, practice is required for fast, accurate implanting.

The point of the needle should be inserted approximately 1/2 to 1 1/2 in. from the base of the ear. The

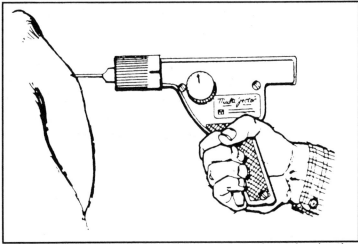

TRICKY NEEDLE WORK. Experience from implanting many thousands of cattle shows that the maximum growth response comes from properly implanting these pellets. In this way, drug release is sustained over a 60 to 120 day period rather than being absorbed too rapidly or not at all.

skin in this area is relatively loose; further from the base of the ear, the skin becomes much tighter and insertion of the needle is more difficult. The implant site may be above or below the midline of the ear. Use whichever implant site is easier for the operator.

After the needle is inserted, the point should be directed to the middle of the ear. It should be possible to feel the point of the needle under the skin. As the trigger of the implant gun is squeezed, the operator should be able to feel the pellets as they are expelled from the needle. If there is resistance, it is likely the cartilage has been gouged and the pellets may be crushed. Crushed pellets foul the needle and may render the implanting gun inoperable.

Experience from implanting thousands of cattle indicates maximum growth response is observed when pellets are properly implanted. Drug release is sustained over a period of time (60-120 days) rather than being absorbed too fast or not being absorbed at all.

In summary, response to implanted growth-stimulating drugs is a result of sustained release and absorption from the implant site. Careful implanting technique will increase rate of gain, improve feed conversion and lower your cost of gain.

Chapter 29

Trimming Your Cattle Shipping Losses

TRUCK OVERCROWDING is perhaps the most common cause of cattle marketing losses. Losses running into millions of dollars are suffered each year as a result of unnecessarily damaged carcasses due to poor trucking practices.

Stockmen generally are not aware of the high losses caused by bruises, since such injuries are determined after slaughter.

The producer usually has his check by the time the animal is slaughtered and he thinks the loss is the packers'. However, packers have learned through experience the percent of such losses and these deductions are reflected in the prices bid for live animals before the producer ever gets his check.

Most bruised carcasses result from horn damage, careless handling, overcrowding, prodding with clubs or obstacles found in the feedlot.

Prevent Costly Losses

Most damage could be prevented by dehorning, careful handling with proper loading ramps, using canvas slappers instead of clubs and by careful loading.

The floor of the truck should be sanded to a depth

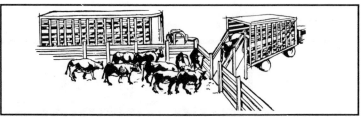

TREAT 'EM RIGHT! If you take the time to properly handle your beef animals during shipping, it will pay big dividends.

of 3 to 4 in. to give cattle a good footing and to prevent them from slipping. On long hauls to market or in cold weather, it is also advisable to place a layer of straw 12 to 18 in. deep on top of the sand.

With numerous sized trucks available, a cattle producer should have no trouble securing the right size to accommodate his shipment of animals to market. When too many cattle are crowded into a truck, they may get along all right until one lies down or is jerked down by a sudden stop or movement. In many cases, this animal is never able to regain its feet and is trampled by the other animals all the way to market.

Beef carcass damage losses are usually hidden, but they also can be easily controlled to a great extent.

Shrink Is A Big Concern

The single biggest loss every livestock producer suffers is shrink. Experts agree that most shrink occurs in the first one quarter of the distance to be traveled and is due largely to fear and excitement.

Handle livestock slowly and make them as comfortable as possible during their ride. Keep them cool in summer and draft-free in the winter. It means extra money in your pocket.

Chapter 30

Using Your Dairy Cow Record Sheets

WHEN IT COMES to being a top-notch dairy manager, nothing beats having a good set of production, breeding and health records for ready reference. In fact, you need this kind of information on hand at all times to be an effective dairy manager.

You may keep this information on two-sided record forms, such as those shown in this chapter which are offered by the publishers of this book. Or you may utilize a computer system to store this data. The important thing is to use whatever record keeping method works best for you.

Here's a rundown on the type of valuable information you should be faithfully keeping on all of your dairy animals:

Sketch Or Photograph All Animals

As soon as a dairy cow, heifer or calf enters your herd, be sure to properly record her identity. Either take a snapshot or carefully sketch the color markings of the animal's left and right sides and head on a card for each animal. This will provide positive identification of the animal when all other means of identification, such as ear tags, chains, etc., are somehow lost.

Sketching is a relatively easy job, even though it

may seem extremely difficult for the beginner to do. One suggestion might be to have your wife or daughter handle the sketching work for you—in most instances, they are rather good at it.

Should You Name Your Cows?

In a smaller dairy herd, there are many advantages to giving each cow a name instead of trying to simply identify her by ear tag number, neck chain, stanchion in the barn or some other method.

Some major advantages to naming your cows:

☞ It is quicker and easier to remember a name than a complicated ear tag or chain number. Even though breeding work requires that you check the ear tag or sketch carefully for positive identification, a name is usually enough to identify the animal in the barn.

☞ Names are better to use than a number in a stanchion barn because you can move the animal from one stanchion to another without causing a mix-up in your records. Memory is generally a poor record of such changes and can cause mistakes.

☞ Names are also easier to follow through most of the records that you will keep.

☞ It is important that you use the same name for only one cow to keep the records straight. Putting 2nd, 3rd, etc. behind a name for calves from a certain cow isn't much better than using stanchion numbers since it will only lead to confusion. For additional help in naming purebred cows eligible for registry, write to your breed association.

Using The Cow's Own Name

The name of the cow can also be helpful to the dairyman in other ways than simply for identification. To be able to know the sire and age of the cow just from the animal's name, follow these simple steps:

If your animal is a purebred that is eligible for registration with the breed association, you may want to use a "prefix"—a word that identifies all animals bred on your farm which is always the first word in the animal's registered name.

This "prefix" will be registered by your breed association after they have checked to see that no one else in the entire country has registered it first. Your prefix may even be the first name of your farm.

If your cow is a grade animal, use the barn name of the cow's sire as the first name. This will tell you who sired the animal whenever you look at her name.

Follow this first name with a feminine name which is coded for the animal's age. For example, use "A" as the beginning letter for the name of every animal born in 1991, "B" to start the name for those born in 1992, etc. A calf born in 1991 and sired by Stonehill Butter-King Rocket might be named *Rocket* (barn name of sire) *Ada* (this second name tells us the female animal was born in 1991).

A calf from the same cow and sired by the same bull in 1992 might be named *Rocket Beth* (the "B" in Beth indicates a heifer born in 1992 while Rocket indicates the bull that fathered the calf).

If you wish to use a prefix (usually your farm name or your own name), this would be added at the beginning of the calves' names. Using Sunnylawn as a example you would use:

- *Sunnylawn Rocket Ada* for an animal which was born in 1991.

- *Sunnylawn Rocket Beth* for an animal which was born in 1992.

In addition to the cow's name, it is also wise to record the ear tag number and chain number if the cow has a neck chain. This will give you extra methods of identification in all cases.

Critical Information To Record

In addition to proper identification by sketching, name, ear tag and chain numbers, the date the animal was born as well as the sire and dam of the cow will often prove to be very valuable in breeding and managing the cow. This information will quickly give you the cow's age and breeding history so you know when to breed her and what sire to use. This is especially important if the naming system explained earlier is not used.

Milk Production Records

Year-by-year milk production records will prove very valuable when selling cows and their offspring. They are also very valuable for selecting calves for your own herd from the best producing cows. They can also be used as one factor in carrying out a culling program for your dairy herd.

FRONT OF DAIRY CARD. This side of the record card provides room for recording essential information dealing with identification, milk production and a breeding history.

Breeding Records

Good breeding records are very important to any good herd manager. Such information will help you determine when to breed and when to expect the cow to freshen, as well as provide complete data on the new calf. You should record data on the date bred, bull used, date due, date calved and pertinent information on the resulting calf.

Disease, Health History

So you may have a complete and compact record on each cow, a disease and health history section for each animal is included on the back of the card. This history can prove very valuable to both you and your veterinarian. Since it is hard to remember this information accurately over several years, you

Disease & Health History

Date	Symptoms	Diagnosed As	Results

Disposal of Cow (Date & Reason) _____

BACK OF DAIRY CARD. This side of the card contains considerable space for documenting a disease and health history for each animal. There's room for dates, disease and health symptoms, diagnosis, treatments and results.

will always know the date, symptoms, diagnosis and result of the illness when you write it down on these handy record forms.

Good Records Earn Big Dividends

Good records are only be as good as you make them. Use these handy forms for both convenience and help in properly managing your dairy herd.

Chapter 31

Dairy Herd Diseases And Management

A DAIRY HERD health program should include a well thought-out immunization program to prevent disease before it occurs. A good immunization program ensures the dairy cow against many diseases.

Not all diseases can be prevented by vaccination, but many important diseases are preventable by following a well thought-out immunization schedule. The effectiveness of an immunization procedure depends upon the care and administration of the biologics used along with the age and health of the animal at the time of vaccination.

Immunization Schedules

In general, strong disease protection cannot be obtained by vaccinating a calf under 2 months of age. The exception is brucellosis, for which heifer replacements should be vaccinated between 2 and 6 months of age. If other vaccines are used, the calf should be vaccinated at 4 to 6 months of age.

2 To 6 Months Of Age

Administer strain 19 vaccine for essential brucellosis protection.

4 To 6 Months Of Age

Any of the following biologic products can be administered to calves at this age: Infectious Bovine Rhinotracheitis, Parainfluenza, Clostridial group, Haemophilus somnus, BRSV, Bovine Respiratory Syncytial Virus, Bovine Virus Diarrhea (administer this last vaccine 2 weeks after those listed above unless it is of the killed type). Killed virus products are preferred.

13 Months Of Age—2 Months Before Breeding

Give Leptospirosis (five serotypes) and Vibriosis (if natural service is used). Repeat Infectious Bovine Rhinotracheitis. Repeat BVD vaccine, killed preferred, BRSV and Haemophilus somnus vaccine.

Mature Cow—1 Month Before Breeding

Administer booster vaccinations, Leptospirosis, Vibriosis (if natural service is used), IBR (Infectious Bovine Rhinotracheitis), BVD (Bovine Virus Diarrhea) and E. coli.

Follow your veterinarian's recommendation on the selection, use and administration of all biologics.

The successful dairyman has a dairy herd health program in operation which is carefully monitored by his veterinarian.

Proper Analysis Of Your Dairy Herd

A thorough analysis is essential using all existing records which are available. They should include production records, nutrition program, facilities, immunization program, calf raising program, milking machine function, milking technique, udder health program and cost of milk production. An effective and successful record keeping system is absolutely essential.

Goals Must Be Established, Achieved

You, your dairy farm workers and your veterinarian must all work together closely to develop a successful herd health program and to make sure that all aspects of it are carried out.

Your Role As A Dairyman

Here's what you as a dairy producer should do to have a successful dairy health program:

- Two heat cycles by 60 days postpartum.

- Average of 60 days to first service.

- Less than two services per conception.

- No cows open over 100 days without a heat period.

- Average days open and not bred—100 days.

- Less than 10% incidence of retained placenta.

- Less than 10% incidence of metritis.

- Less than 5% incidence of abortion.

- Less than 5% cows culled because of reproduction problems.

- Less than 15% of cows with mastitis during lactation.

- Less than 5% mortality in calves.

- Cost of milk production should be less than $10.00 per cwt.

- Your rolling herd average should be over 15,000 lbs. of milk.

Your Veterinarian's Role

At the same time, here's what your veterinarian should be providing you with a customized dairy health program:

- Conduct monthly or semi-monthly reproductive checks.

- Set up herd immunization program.

- Set up mastitis control program.

- Analyze and adjust rations.

- Check milking machine function.

- Implement a successful calf survival program.

- Make your dairy herd more profitable.

Two Optional Calf Health Programs

Your goal should be to develop a protected calf that will go into the milking herd immunized with the recommended biologics. Then annual booster inoculations can be given after the cow freshens.

Depending on your previous dairy herd health management program, you will want to take a look at the following two options.

1 The following is a program to use if no previous immunization program has been used in your dairy herd in the past:

Open Heifers, Cows—30 Days After Calving

IBR (Infectious Bovine Rhinotracheitis).

PI3 (Parainfluenza).

Haemophilus somnus.

Leptospirosis (Lepto)—Select a vaccine that contains five different leptospira antigens. (Use vibrio vaccine at this time only if a natural mating service is being used).

BVD (Bovine Virus Diarrhea)—Administer 2 weeks after the administration of other vaccines. At this time, also give a booster shot of H. somnus.

Killed BVD vaccine can be used at any time, even for pregnant cows. Two injections, 2 weeks apart, are recommended.

Calves—1 Day To 3 Months

IBR.

PI3.

Pasteurella (This type of health protection for calves is not recommended by all veterinarians).

Haemophilus.

Clostridial group (all seven antigens).

Two Weeks Later

BVD (modified live or killed).

Booster inoculations of H. somnus and Pasteurella. This should be repeated when calves are 4 to 6 months of age.

Calves—4 to 6 Months Of Age

Follow the same program as outlined for younger calves.

Open Heifers

Some 40 to 60 days prior to the first breeding date, administer IBR, PI3, BVD, Lepto and Vibrio (if natural mating is used).

2 The following is the health treatment system you should follow in your herd if an immunization program has been in effect with young dairy calves:

Lactating Herd

Administer IBR, PI3, BVD and Lepto 30 days after calving.

Open Heifers—40 to 60 Days Prior To First Breeding Date

Administer IBR, PI3, H. somnus and Pasteurella.

Calves—3 to 6 Months Of Age

Give shots of IBR, PI3, H. somnus and Pasteurella.

Two Weeks Later

Give BVD and booster inoculations of H. somnus and Pasteurella.

Calves Under 3 Months Of Age

No immunizations are required at this stage unless specific health problems exist with your calves.

Specific Vaccines

Use E. coli bacterin K99 antigen for the prevention of enteritis in the newborn calf due to E. coli infections. Administer two injections to all pregnant cows at 6 and 3 weeks prior to calving.

Reovirus (Rotavirus) and Coronovirus vaccines also can be used in the pregnant cow prior to calving. They will prevent enteritis in the newborn calf due to these viral agents.

Administer strain 19 (Brucellosis) to all heifers (not to bulls) between the ages of 2 and 6 months.

Immunization Precautions

Do not vaccinate pregnant cows with modified live vaccines unless an outbreak of a virus infection exists within the herd.

Do not use modified live BVD vaccine in stressed animals. Administer modified live BVD vaccine 2 weeks after IBR and PI3 have been given. Killed BVD vaccine can be used at any time. At this time, administer booster inoculations of H. somnus and Pasteurella. (Single injections of Pasteurella and H. somnus do not give desirable protection.) Do not administer Strain 19 (Brucellosis) with other vaccines as shock may occur.

Check with your veterinarian relative to all of these health management recommendations. Specific problems in individual dairy herds may significantly alter these recommendations.

Chapter 32

Dairy Disease
Trouble Shooting Guide

THESE PRACTICAL management ideas can help you prevent and treat disease problems in your dairy herd.

Mastitis

This includes Streptococcus ssp., Staphylococci ssp., E. coli and several other types of infectious organisms.

Signs: Increase in somatic cell count. Abnormal milk. Swelling and a fever in toxic animals.

Prevention: Follow a complete program. Use Somato-Staph for prevention of Staph ssp. infections. Use teat dipping after milking and dry cow treatment for all infected udder quarters.

Treatment: The best program to follow will depend on the type of organism involved and sensitivity testing. Intramammary or intravenous routes give best results. Oral feeding of drugs is not recommended. If needed, feed zinc methionine at at rate of 2 grams per head per day or 1 lb. per 495 lbs. of bodyweight per day.

Drug Withholding Period: Withhold milk from market for 96 hours after treatment. Withhold treated cows from slaughter for 30 days.

Cowpox Virus

Signs: Sensitive teats and udder. Lesions start out as a papule and then become a vesicle, followed by a pustule and scab.

Prevention: There is no treatment that will destroy this virus. Avoid bringing the virus in with any new herd replacements.

Do not use a sponge when washing udders. Use a recommended teat dip after milking.

Treatment: Use antibiotic ointments after milking to keep down secondary infections.

Drug Withholding Period: None.

Winter Dysentery

This disease is probably caused by a virus, although it has never been isolated.

Signs: Diarrhea lasting for 3-6 days, usually in stanchioned herds.

Prevention: Treatment must be differentiated from the treatments for Virus Diarrhea, Coccidiosis and Salmonellosis.

Treatment: Sulfonamides or Antibiotics. Check with your veterinarian.

Drug Withdrawal Period: Check with your local veterinarian.

Ketosis (Metabolic)

Signs: Cattle go off feed and milk production drops.

Prevention: Feed propylene glycol at a rate of 1/4 to 1/2 lb. per head per day beginning 2 weeks after freshening. Continue for 6 weeks. Sodium propionate can also be fed twice daily continuously for 6 weeks after calving.

Treatment: Proplyene glycol fed at a rate of 1/4 to 1 lb. (4 to 16 fluid oz.) per head per day for 10 days or feed sodium propionate at a rate of 1/2 lb. twice daily for 10 days. Check with your veterinarian.

Drug Withholding Period: None.

Colibacillosis (E. coli)

Signs: Enteritis in newborn animals.

Prevention: Vaccinate cows twice within a 30-day period prior to calving with E. coli vaccine containing K99 antigen. The calf must obtain dam's colostrum milk at birth or be given a genetically engineered vaccine immediately after birth.

Treatment: Electrolytes and antibiotics.

Drug Withdrawal Period: None

Milk Fever (Metabolic)

Signs: A lack of coordination in your dairy cattle. Animals may be down before or after freshening.

Prevention: 20 million units of vitamin D2 administered each day in two equal feedings for 5 to 7 days before calving.

Treatment: Calcium products in an intravenous injection.

Drug Withholding Period: None.

Grass Tetany (Hypomagnesemia)

Signs: Nervousness, staggering, convulsions and death in dairy animals.

Prevention: This problem usually occurs on fresh, succulent, well-fertilized forage. Feed magnesium oxide at a rate of 1/2 to 1 oz. per head per day.

Treatment: Administer magnesium sulfate in an IV at 200 ml of 25% solution.

Drug Withholding Period: None.

Johne's Disease

These disease problems can include Paratuberculosis or Mycobacterium. A laboratory confirmation is necessary.

Signs: Chronic diarrhea.

Prevention: A vaccine is available in some states. Test and remove all reactors. Develop a hygenic program for calves which should be separated from the adult dairy herd.

Treatment: Temporary treatment can come from symptomatic treatment, but there is no complete cure.

Drug Withholding Period: None.

Vibriosis (Vibrio Fetus)

Signs: Repeat breeding services.

Prevention: Vaccinate females and bulls prior to breedings. Use artificial insemination with tested bulls to prevent the disease. Use untried bulls only on virgin heifers.

Treatment: None.

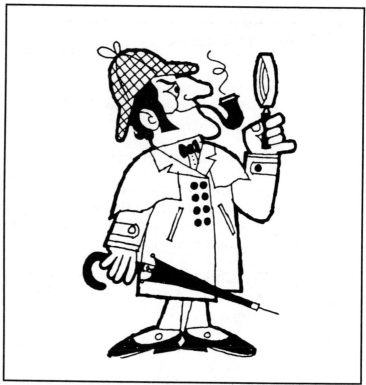

KNOW CRITICAL DAIRY DISEASE SYMPTOMS. Carefully study information on the most important diseases outlined in this chapter that commonly affect dairy herds.

Leukosis

The cause of this disease is not known, but a virus is suspected. Laboratory diagnosis is necessary.

Signs: Enlarged lymph nodes.

Prevention: Prohibit the sale of animals with this disease for breeding purposes. Prevent all infected animals from going into non-infected herds.

Treatment: None.

Chapter 33

Controlling Internal Parasites In Dairy Cattle

A NUMBER of internal parasites can have a very drastic influence on production in your dairy herd.

Cattle Dewormers

There are several dewormers on the market which are very effective. They are available as boluses, feed additives, drench and injectable forms.

Available dewormers are Levamisole (Tramisol), Phenothiazine, Thiabendazole, Fenbendazole,

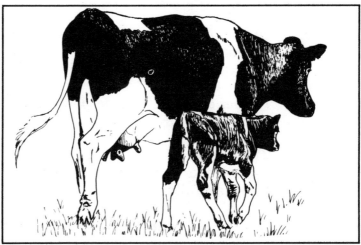

AVOID COSTLY LOSSES. When it comes to selecting a dewormer, you have a variety of products to choose from.

Safe Guard or Pancur, Ivermectin, Valbazen, Coumaphas (for lactating dairy cows where the milk can be sold) and Morantel tartrate. All these products are efficacious for most species of worms. However, some of these products have a broader spectrum than others.

Worm loads, types of worms found in different geographical areas and preferred forms of dewormers for administration will all dictate your dewormer of choice. Veterinarians familiar with your herd and with the aid of fecal examinations can assist cattlemen in the proper choice of dewormers and their frequency of use.

Since all cattle possess worm parasites, they should be placed on a scheduled worming procedure.

Gastrol Intestinal

This category includes all types of these parasites and lungworms.

Signs: Anemia, unthriftiness, feed utilization and weight gains can be affected. Internal parasitism is frequently not clinically detected.

Prevention: Strategic deworming is needed to prevent pasture contamination.

Treatment: Several different dewormers can be used. Check with your veterinarian and read the label carefully.

Drug Withholding Period: Check dewormer labels as withdrawal periods can range from 2 to 8 days.

Cysticerosis (Beef measles)

This can result in an invasion of muscles by beef tapeworm in man (Taenia saginata).

Signs: No symptoms are normally found on post-mortem.

Prevention: Keep dogs and your cow herd out of feedlots.

Treatment: None.

Echinococcosis

Cysts are caused by dog tapeworm. This can be a public health hazard.

Signs: No symptoms are usually found on post-mortem.

Prevention: Keep dogs out of feedlots.

Treatment: None.

Coccidiosis

This is a major disease problem in young beef and dairy cattle. It frequently is not treated until it becomes an acute problem.

Signs: Diarrhea, solid tailhead and blood-tinged feces.

Prevention: Use clean, dry pens. Avoid stress in your young animals. Add Decoquinate (Decox at a rate of 0.5 mg. per kilogram of bodyweight for 28 to 150 days) and Amprolium to the ration at a rate of 5 mg. per kilogram of bodyweight for 21 days..

Treatment: Feed Decoquinate at a rate of 10 mg per kilogram of bodyweight for 5 days or Amprolium at a rate of 10 mg per kilogram of bodyweight for 5 days.

Drug Withholding Period: None.

Chapter 34

Properly Managing Dairy Reproduction

GETTING THE COW with calf is one of the most important parts of any herd health program. A separate record system is often needed.

There are a number of record systems available that include animal identification, heat dates, breeding dates, pregnancy determination, treatments and date of calving. The system must be simple and need not be expensive. Such record keeping forms can be obtained from the Cooperative Extension Service, breed associations, A.I. stud services and the publishers of this book.

"Mathematical factors" to use in herd reproduction include:

- A—Heat (estrus) detection.

- B—Cow fertility.

- C—Bull fertility.

- D—Timing of insemination or mating and/or technique.

- E—Disease status and calving problems.

The resulting equation for a live, healthy calf is A x B x C x D x E equals a live calf. If any factor is zero, the product is "zero calf."

Goals And Guidelines

The breeding goals for any dairy herd, regardless of its size, should be:

Days open—50 to 75 days.

Inseminations per conception—1.5 to 1.8.

Total inseminations—1.85.

Days to first insemination—35 to 55 days.

Breed heifers—13 months of age.

A good reproductive management program includes the following guidelines for reproductive tract examination. These examinations should be done by a veterinarian on a regularly scheduled basis:

1 Examine all cows at least once after calving (14 to 28 days after calving) for rate of involution and vaccinate for IBR, PI3, BVD and Lepto.

2 Re-examine and continue to examine cows with abnormal involutions until they are ready for rebreeding.

3 Examine all cows who are fresh 60 days or longer and not yet showing heat.

4 Examine all cows bred three or more times. Re-examine them after the next breeding.

5 Examine all cows with abnormal heat cycles at the time of breeding.

6 Examine all cows with abnormal vaginal discharges and treat accordingly.

7 Examine all cows bred 30 days or more to see if they are pregnant.

An accurate, up-to-date record keeping system is essential to keep track of each cow's reproductive status and treatments.

Proper Heat Detection

In a study of sterility and delayed breeding in dairy cattle, New York researchers found 75% of the breeding problems were due to management faults. The most important job on a dairy farm is heat detection. It is for that reason that a review of the heat cycle and its associated signs is presented here.

When a cow comes into heat (estrus) a follicle, which is the egg-bearing structure, develops on the ovary. This follicle is stimulated to development by the Follicle Stimulating Hormone (FSH) which is secreted by the pituitary and carried to the ovary through the blood stream. Once the follicle develops, the cow is in heat. Estrogens (hormones) are then released via the bloodstream that affect the pituitary gland by stopping the secretion of FSH and stimulating a Luteinizing Hormone (LH).

When there is a certain amount of LH and FSH in the bloodstream, ovulation occurs and the egg is

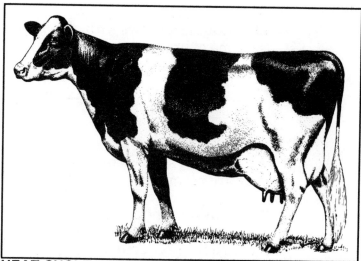

HEAT CYCLE. The follicle stimulating hormone released by the pituitary gland causes the egg to develop. This follicle contains estrogen which helps promotes heat. When the follicle stimulating hormone is no longer released, luteinizing hormone causes the follicle to rupture. Progesterone is needed for the maintenance of pregnancy.

released into the fallopian tube. The hormone LH stimulates the pit or depression to be filled with tissue called the corpus luteum (yellow body). This in turn produces a hormone called progesterone which is necessary for the maintenance of pregnancy. If pregnancy does not occur, the corpus luteum decreases in size, progesterone levels decrease and FSH takes over again to bring about another estrous cycle.

The cow has two ovaries and they do not necessarily alternate in their 21-to 22-day rhythmic cycles.

After it is shed into the fallopian tube, the egg moves slowly and does not reach the uterus for 70 to 90 hours. It is within the fallopian tube that the sperm meets the egg and fertilization takes place. Sperm transport from the area of deposition (ante-

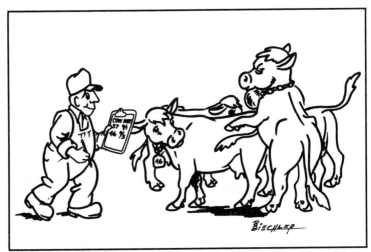

HEAT CYCLE REVIEW. Make sure you understand how the heat cycle works with your dairy animals and the key signs associated with it. This is crucial to your success as 75% of breeding problems are due to management faults.

rior cervix) to the point of fertilization, varies in time. Sperm transport is most rapid from the middle to the end of the heat period, taking a few minutes to 2 or 3 hours, depending upon the stage of the estrus (heat).

The fertilized egg does not immediately attach to the uterine wall after it enters the uterine horn. It remains unattached for 30 to 50 days. However, the fetal membranes are rapidly developing and may extend into the nonpregnant uterine horn by the time attachment takes place.

Various Signs Of Heat

The average cow comes into heat every 21 days, but there is a range from 18 to 24 days. The time interval between estrus periods is constant in the normal cow.

Most cows stay in heat around 18 hours, but the range is from 6 to 36 hours. Early in the estrus period the cow shows nervousness, decreased milk flow and swelling of the vulvar lips. After the nervous signs are exhibited, the cow shows a willingness to accept the bull, a period called "standing heat."

The average cow is in standing heat for 6 to 15 hours, perhaps longer if not serviced by the bull. Ovulation, when the egg is dropped, always occurs 7 to 12 hours after estrus. As a result, the correct time to breed a cow is near the end of her estrus period regardless of the length of the period, because sperm normally live only 12 to 24 hours in the reproductive tract.

During the estrus period, there is an increased blood supply to the reproductive tract, resulting in the rupture of a few small vessels. A small amount of blood is liberated and is observed passing from the reproductive tract 12 to 24 hours after the estrus period. This is no indication that the cow has or has not settled. It is observed in 80% to 85% of cows. Frequently, pregnant cows will still come into heat.

Signs Of Coming In Heat

As a cow begins to come in heat she shows the following signs and symptoms in the 8 hours previous to standing heat:

1 Bawling more than normal.

2 Leaves herd and walks a fence in an attempt to get into adjoining pastures with other cattle.

3 Attempts to mount or ride other animals.

4 Tail is wet near vulva.

5 Vulva is slightly swollen, moist and red.

6 Smells rear end of other cows.

7 Will not usually stand to be ridden by other cows.

8 May have a clear mucous discharge from vulva.

9 Is usually down in milk production.

10 Fails to eat normally.

Signs Of Standing Heat

When in standing heat (usually about 18 hours), a cow or heifer will show some of the following characteristics:

☞ Stands to be ridden.

☞ Will ride other cows.

☞ Bawls frequently.

☞ Nervous and excitable.

☞ Usually down in milk production.

☞ Off-feed or refuses to eat.

When a cow is going out of heat (usually over a 12-hour period) she will act as follows:

• Will not stand to be ridden by other cows.

• Will attempt to ride other cows.

• Smells other cows.

• Up in milk production.

• Appetite normal, eats normally.

• May have clear mucous discharge from vulva.

The second day after heat ends, a slight bloody discharge will be noticed. When heat was not detected (silent heat) but this symptom was noticed, the cow should be in heat 16 to 19 days later. This

---

How To Spot Physical Signs Of Heat

Coming Into Heat—8 Hours

1. Stands and bellows.
2. Smells other cows.
3. Attempts to ride other cows, but will not stand.
4. Vulva is moist, red and slightly swollen.
5. May have clear mucous discharge from vulva.

Standing Heat—18 Hours
1. Stands to be ridden.
2. Bellows frequently.
3. Nervous and excitable.
4. Rides other cows.
5. Best time to breed is during the middle to end of this period.

Going Out Of Heat
1. Will not stand to be ridden, but attempts to mount.
2. Smells other cows.
3. May have clear mucous discharge from vulva.

---

is a very fine point but an excellent symptom for the herdsman to look for in some cows.

The discharging of blood by the cow or heifer is a normal occurrence and is probably due to the breakdown of some of the cells which line the uterus.

Abnormal Heat

Normally, cows come into estrus within 18 to 24 days from the last recorded heat period. Heat periods falling outside these ranges (16 days or less and 24 days or more) should be regarded with suspicion and considered abnormal. The veterinarian will be most interested in abnormally short, long, or irregular heat cycles because such information is useful relative to the treatment of a specific cow.

Factors Affecting Heat

The following factors may affect heat periods in a low percentage of the cows within a herd:

Length Of Heat Period In The Dairy Cow (Standing Heat)

No. Of Hours	Cows	% Of Total
1-3	1	0.8
4-6	3	2.3
7-9	4	3.0
10-12	17	12.1
13-15	26	20.5
16-18	32	24.3
19-21	25	18.9
22-24	18	13.6
25-27	4	3.0
28-30	2	1.5

—Pennsylvania State Univ.

**Length Of Time Between
End Of Heat And Ovulation**

No. Of Hours	Cows	% Of Total
3-4	5	3.8
5-6	9	6.8
7-8	24	18.2
9-10	29	21.9
11-12	36	27.3
13-14	19	14.4
15-16	7	5.3

—Pennsylvania State Univ.

- The cow may be pregnant.

- The uterus may contain an infection. Uterine infections will prevent the occurrence of heat.

- There may be a cyst in the corpus luteum (yellow body). This usually occurs after calving.

- Extremely high temperatures (95 to 105 degrees F.) affect the length of the heat period.

- Cows under heavy stress—high production, heat stress, anemia, infection—will not show evidence of heat.

- Heifers on a low level of nutrition will not show heat. For example, a phosphorous deficiency may prevent heat.

Remember that over 90% of cows that are reported not to be in heat have been missed by the dairyman.

About 80% of all heat periods will show a duration

of 15 to 18 hours. See details in the table shown here.

Ovulation or the release of the ovum from the ovarian follicle occurs 10 to 17 hours after the termination of heat or estrus.

The cooperation of both the dairyman and the technician is essential to get a desirable non-return rate. Following a few thumb rules will result in satisfactory breeding performance.

Cows that are found in heat in the morning should be bred during the afternoon of the same day. Cows that are found in heat after 10 a.m. should be bred the next morning.

In instances where dairymen have both an a.m. cow in heat and a p.m. cow from the previous day, the technician should make every effort to arrive at that farm in the middle of the day so as to breed both cows at one time.

Exceptions to these rules are small percentages of the cow population with either abnormally long or short intervals from the onset of estrus until ovulation. As cows tend to repeat the same kind of heat periods, it is necessary to make proper allowances for these cows.

While timing of insemination is critical for conception there may be other reasons why cows don't settle:

- Failure to ovulate.

- Hormone imbalance.

- Fertilization does not take place.

- Low quality semen.

- Poor nutrition.

During a typical estrous cycle, ovulation takes place about 25 to 30 hours after the onset of estrus. It has been determined by experimentation that motile and non-motile spermatozoa are transported to the ovarian end of the fallopian within 2 1/2 to 10 minutes following insemination. It is in this region of the fallopian tube that fertilization of the ovum by the sperm occurs.

The length of time that sperm and ova remain fertile in the reproductive tract of the cow is not exactly known. It is believed that an ovum is fertile for only a few hours after it is released from the

Influence Of Timing On Conception Rate*

Time Of Service (Before Or After Heat)	Cows	% Conception
18-12 hrs before	25	44.0
12-6 hrs before	40	82.5
6-0 hrs before	40	75.0
0-6 hrs after	40	62.5
6-12 hrs after	25	32.0
12-18 hrs after	25	28.0
12-24 hrs after	25	12.0

Egg will live 6 to 10 hours in reproductive tract; 6 hours required for sperm capacitation.

—Univ. of Wisconsin

Critical Days Lost
Between Pregnancies*

Reason	Days Lost**	Percent
Unsuccessful service	19.1	45.3
Missed estrus	17.9	42.5
Cystic ovaries	2.1	5.0
Abortion (34-150 days)	2.1	5.0
Uterine infection	0.4	1.0
Abnormal reproductive tract	0.3	0.7
Abortion (151-230 days)	0.2	0.5

*884 cows
**Cows losing over 100 days.
—North Carolina State Univ.

ovary of the cow or heifer.

Sperm remain fertile over longer periods of time. Estimates of 24 to 30 hours have been given for the upper limit. Consequently, if conception is to occur, insemination and ovulation must coincide within the limits of the range of fertilization of the germ cells. Because these fundamental physiological factors do exist, it has been generally recommended that the correct time to breed a cow is at or near the end of her heat period.

There is no doubt that a latitude of several hours

exists in obtaining the optimum time to breed a cow. Certainly the chance for conception is better if the semen is deposited in the uterus within 12 hours of ovulation rather than 25 to 30 hours prior to ovulation which is the case when the cow is bred at the onset of estrus. In nature, the bull takes care of these physiological factors by breeding the cow as long as she is in standing heat.

Heat Detection

This is the real key to obtaining a high conception rate in your dairy herd. Heat detection is the most difficult task in maximizing A.I. usage. While cows in most herds cycle in a normal, regular pattern, detecting and recording all heat periods is needed to help identify the problem cows.

Heat detection requires time and patience and cannot be relegated to one not familiar with the behavior of a cow during different phases of her estrous cycle.

Checking for heat should be done three times a day—morning, midday and in the evening. Research has shown that approximately 90% of so-called "heat failure" detections are due to the dairyman and not the cow herself.

Most cows come into heat during the night. Almost half the cows first exhibit estrus in the morning and are not in estrus by evening. For this reason, cows should be checked for estrus as close to dark and as close to dawn as possible.

Idaho studies have shown that if a herd is checked for heat only twice a day then 27% of all the heat periods will go undetected. Louisiana workers found that by observing the herd (plus breeding heifers) four times a day at equal intervals, two-thirds of the missed heats can be detected. Thus the value of management is again shown as the key to catching cows in heat.

North Carolina studies have shown 42 1/2% of the days lost between pregnancies are due to missed (undetected heats) estrus periods.

False Heats

With false heats, between 5% and 10% of pregnant heifers and cows will exhibit heat symptoms, even up to the point of "heavy springer" heifers. If such animals have been diagnosed and declared pregnant, then these heats should be recorded but the cow should not be bred.

If an insemination tube is passed through the cervix of a cow safe in calf (pregnant), an abortion will surely occur. A herdsmen should be alert for false heats.

Heat Detection Aids

Heat detection aids are excellent helping hands when cows are hard to "catch in heat." All heat detection aids must be strongly supplemented with close visual observation by you or your employees on a regular basis.

Teaser or gomer bulls fitted with chin-ball markers have also been used with success. Surgical penile deflection coupled with partial epididymectomy or

vasectomy has been more successful than penec-
tomy or penile blocks.

Steers, cows and heifers injected with testosterone
can be induced to serve as detectors in beef and
dairy herds. Injections of 500 mg of testosterone
propionate in oil given intramuscularly on days
one, five and ten will induce most animals to serve
as detectors when equipped with a chin-ball harness. A booster injection is recommended 2 to 3
weeks later. Detector animals must be structurally
sound and weigh 700 to 800 lbs.

Chin-ball marking devices must be properly fitted.
An empty harness should be put on the detector for
3 or 4 days prior to use as a detector animal. The
reservoir should be filled when the teaser is added
to the herd and checked every 5 days. Different
colored fluids can be used if more than one bull is
used. No more than 30 females per animal detector
is recommended.

Female identification is necessary. Hot brands,
cold brands, neck chains or ear tags should be used.

Handling Cows In Heat

During estrus, all cows and heifers (of breeding
age) should be confined in individual pens with
water and forage (hay, silage, etc.) available. All
heat dates should be recorded at a specific place in
the dairy office that is agreed upon by the herdsman, milkers, the A.I. technician and veterinarian.

There should not be any compromise on this management principle whatsoever, as the chance for
success in our herd's overall breeding efficiency is
decreased.

```
        Relationship Of Days Open
        To Services Per Conception

Days Open          Services Per Conception*
30                 2.50
40                 2.25
50                 2.05
60                 1.85
70                 1.75
```

It is estimated that an extra 0.2 straws of semen will be needed per cow in a herd having a voluntary waiting period of 40 days compared to a waiting period of 60 days.

—*Ohio State Univ.*

Rebreeding Cows

When is a cow's reproductive tract ready for breeding? A 60-day waiting period between calving and rebreeding has long been a recommended practice. But recent research indicates this rest period is not necessary.

Considerable time can be saved if the cow is bred at the first heat after 35 to 40 days postpartum. Calving intervals can be shortened by approximately 15 days by reducing the waiting period by 20 days. Five days are lost due to missed heats and a slightly lower conception rate. Services required per conception estimated at various days open are shown in the table here.

The slightly higher semen cost is offset by the

reduced costs which are found with a shorter calving interval. Problems with greater embryonic loss, abortion, metritis, retained placentas or weak calves at birth have not been encountered in several university studies with early dairy rebreeding programs.

In an earlier rebreeding program, around 45% of the cows bred will become pregnant with the first insemination. Since a 40-to 60-day dry period is required for cows to produce at their potential during the next lactation, those conceiving prior to 60 days postpartum, will have lactations shorter than 305 days. This disadvantage is outweighed in most cows, because a greater percentage of their lifetime is spent in peak production which results in increased lifetime milk production.

Reproductive Diseases

There are many abnormal conditions and diseases which can not only lower breeding efficiency, but in extreme cases can lead to milking a herd of open cows. Some of these conditions or diseases include:

1 Cervicitis—inflammation of the cervix.

2 Metritis—inflammation of all uterine tissues.

3 Endometritis—inflammation of uterine lining.

4 Pyometra—accumulation of pus in the uterus which results from untreated endometritis.

5 Vaginitis—inflammation of the vagina.

6 Cystic corpus lutea—cyst of corpus luteum.

7 Non-functioning ovaries.

These conditions can interfere with the normal fertilization process. Proper sanitation of calving facilities, cleanliness when assisting calf delivery and balanced nutrition can reduce the occurrence of these conditions.

While a veterinarian may use intra-uterine infusion for problem cows, it is not recommended for "normal" cows.

A more detailed explanation of diseases known to cause abortion is given at the end of this chapter. Laboratory diagnostic needs, available vaccines and relative abortion times are also given. To lower the incidence of these diseases, use A.I. and raise your own replacements. If you buy replacements, purchase them unbred and breed them artificially.

If bulls must be used, breed virgin heifers to only virgin yearling bulls. This will isolate, identify and perhaps in due time, eliminate disease. Highly infected or older cows may have to be slaughtered in extreme cases to break the chain of infection.

Cost Of Low Fertility*

Herd Size	Expected Yearly Loss**
50	$2,000
70	2,800
100	4,000
200	8,000
300	12,000
500	20,000
1000	40,000

Based on $40 cost per cow per year.
**Losses may be higher if abnormal symptoms are ignored.*

The Cost of Low Fertility

Do your cows calve every 365 days? If not, the following explains why you should maintain a 12-month calving interval:

Compared to a 150 cow herd on a 14 month calving interval, a herd of 125 cows on a 12-month calving interval will:

☛ Produce as much milk.

☛ Produce as many calves for herd replacements.

☛ Require 17% less feed for maintenance.

☛ Require 17% less labor.

☞ Require 17% less barn space and bedding.

☞ Return more net profit per cow.

Low breeding efficiency, along with the labor and mastitis complex, is one of the major problems with

---

DHIA Calving Intervals
(Data from 350 Herds)

Calving Interval	Herds	Breeding Efficiency
11 months	3%	Don't use
12	29%	100%
13	48%	91.7%
14	15.5%	83.3%
15	3%	75.0%
16	1.5%	66.7%

—Univ. Of Georgia

---

which dairymen are confronted. Economic losses in dairy herds amount to over $500 million annually in the U.S. due to reproductive failures.

A dairy cow becomes a reproductive problem if she is not settled (safe in calf) by 100 days after her previous calving. Numerous studies show that it costs dairymen at least $3.00 to $4.00 a day for every day the cow stays open over 100 days. Each time a dairyman has to send a cow to the sale barn due to difficult breeding it costs him about $350 in lost income. This is the difference between an animal's salvage value and the cost of a sound, regular breeding replacement.

Calving Interval

A study of DHIA records shows 68% of the herds had average herd calving intervals ranging from 13 to 16 months. These results point to breeding inefficiency as a dairyman's major problem.

In summary, authorities in the field of reproductive physiology are in general agreement that if our current knowledge and available tools were put to work, at least 75% of current reproductive problems in dairy herds would be prevented or solved.

Diseases Known To Cause Abortion

Here is a more detailed explanation of the key diseases that are known to cause abortion in cattle. Laboratory diagnostic needs, available vaccines, treatments and relative abortion times are also given for each of these critical disease concerns.

Brucellosis

Causative Organism: (Bacterial) Brucella abortus.

Samples Needed For Diagnosis: Blood sample from aborting cow and/or sample from fetus and placenta.

Vaccines Available: Use a live vaccine on Heifers at 2 to 6 months of age.

Time of Abortion: 7-9 months.

Leptospirosis

Causative Organism: Leptospira ssp.

Samples Needed for Diagnosis: two blood samples from aborting cow taken 3 weeks apart. Fetus & placenta samples.

Vaccines Available: Killed vaccine. Immunity is 6-12 months.

Time of Abortion: 7-9 months. Immunity may show up within 6 weeks after infection.

Listeriosis

Causative Organism: Listeria monocyto genes.

Samples Needed for Diagnosis: Fetus and placenta or uterine discharge.

Vaccines Available: None.

Time of Abortion: 6-9 months. Severe metritis is common.

Salmonellosis

Causative Organism: S. typhimurium and S. dublin.

Samples Needed for Diagnosis: Fetus.

Vaccines Available: For some serotypes.

Time of Abortion: 6-9 months. Placenta may be decomposed.

Vibriosis

Causative Organism: Vibrio fetus, var. venerealis or var. intestinalis.

Samples Needed for Diagnosis: Fetus and placenta, Uterine discharge and/or Vaginal mucous.

Vaccines Available: Killed vaccine administered 30-60 days before breeding.

Time of Abortion: Usually 2-6 months.

Trichomoniasis

Causative Organism: Trichomonas Foetus.

Samples Needed for Diagnosis: Fetus and placenta, uterine discharge and/or vaginal mucous.

Vaccines Available: Only one at this time.

Time of Abortion: Usually 2 to 6 months.

Bovine Virus Diarrhea Mucosal Disease

Causative Organism: (Viral) BVD virus.

Samples Needed for Diagnosis: Two blood samples from aborting cow taken 3 weeks apart, fetus and placenta.

Vaccines Available: Modified live virus vaccine and killed virus vaccine.

Time of Abortion: Can occur at anytime, but often occur 4 days to 3 months after an outbreak.

Infectious Bovine Rhinotracheitis (IBR)

Causative Organism: IBR virus.

Samples Needed for Diagnosis: Two blood samples from an aborting cow should be taken 3 weeks apart.

Vaccines Available: Modified live virus vaccine and killed virus vaccine.

Time of Abortion: These can occur at anytime, but they are most likely to happen 4 days to 3 months after an outbreak.

Catarrhal Vaginocervicitis

Causaive Organism: CVC virus.

Samples Needed for Diagnosis: Two blood samples from aborting cow taken 3 weeks apart.

Vaccines Available: None.

Time of Abortion: 5 to 7 months. Stillbirths and mummies can occur.

Chapter 35

Controlling Scours
In Your Dairy Calves

ENTERITIS, commonly called calf scours, is a highly infectious diarrheic disease that is a major cause of losses in newborn calves. Many researchers have felt Escherichia coli is the principal cause.

Causes Of Scours

Many causative agents may actually be involved in causing diarrhea and death in both dairy and beef calves. They include:

- Bacteria-Salmonella dublin, S. derby, S. typhimurium, S. enteritidis, Escherichia coli (over 5,000 serotypes) Proteus, Paracolons, and bacterial toxins (clostridium perfringens, B, C and D).

- Viruses--Rota viruses and corona virus.

- Chlamydia—(PLT).

- Mycoplasma.

- Fungi.

These agents vary in their ability to produce enteritis and in their geographic location. In some sections of the country, a virus may be involved.

Most researchers feel calf scours is a complex disease due to a multiple etiology. The cause of scours usually involves a combination of things such as a susceptible animal, stress, virus, bacteria or other agent.

Susceptible Calves

Some calves may have inherited resistance. Other calves acquire protection from immune bodies found in their dam's colostrum milk. A maximum absorption of this protection occurs within the first 12 to 20 hours of the calf's life.

The calf should receive colostrum immediately after birth before any bacterial action may affect the intestinal tract and produce scours. The dam's colostrum may not contain protective bodies for all causes of scours.

Stress

Chilling, contaminated water and unsanitary lots or shelters all make the calf susceptible to scours.

Bacteria

Evidence is abundant that E. coli and related enteric bacteria are major contributors to the calf scours problem. However, bacteria change constantly in their ability to produce scours; thus, it is nearly impossible to develop immunity in a dam or calf. E. coli causes enteritis in the upper small intestine due to runaway growth in this area which is normally free of coliform bacteria.

Viruses

A number of viruses can cause enteritis or pneumonenteritis in calves. In most experiments, the disease produced by a virus alone is mild. But when coupled with an overwhelming growth of toxin-producing bacteria, the symptoms indicate more severe enteritis.

Management Practices

You can follow a number of proven practices to reduce the impact of scours in your calves.

Calving

Every effort should be made to have the calf born in an environment which is conducive to preventing scours.

Dairy Calves

Clip udder hair. Disinfect the navel immediately after birth with a tie that is placed 1 in. from the body wall. Cut off the remainder and soak the stump in strong tincture of iodine (7%). Sanitize the udder of the cow if she is in a stall. Provide a sanitized, well-bedded maternity stall or calve on pasture.

Move the calf immediately to another building and place it in an individual calf stall. Feed 1 pt. of colostrum immediately. Feed another 1 qt. 12 hours later. Keep a heat lamp over the calf until it is dried off and then maintain room temperature at 55 to 60 degrees. Provide proper ventilation with a forced air system. The building must be dry, so that bedding and surroundings can stay dry.

Beef Calves

Plan your breeding program so calving occurs on pasture instead of mud lots. Or make calving sheds available.

Mixed bacterins are generally believed to be of little value in preventing calf scours.

Heavy milk flow by the dam does not cause scours. However, it may aggravate scours problems that already exist.

If scours develop in a beef calf, begin the following treatment:

- If possible, remove the calf from the cow for 48 hours. Administer scours medicine, but do not feed the calf. After 48 hours, feed sparingly by allowing nursing for 5 to 8 minute periods four times daily.

- If diarrhea persists, continue the treatment for another 48 hours and feed an oral electrolyte solution. A normal nonscouring, non-dehydrated calf needs 30 cc of fluid per pound of body weight per day (example: a 60-lb. calf needs 3 pts. per day).

- If the calf is dehydrated and continues to scour and dehydrate, hospitalize the calf. Place the calf under a heat lamp and have your veterinarian administer fluids containing electrolytes and glucose. A 75 to 100 lb. calf will require 4 to 6 qts. of fluids administered by the drip-method intravenously. Administer these fluids over a 3 to 4 hour period at the rate of 2 cc per pound of body weight per hour.

- If the kidneys are not functioning, the calf will die. If the calf will not drink oral electrolytes, intravenous administration of fluids should be continued. Get 1 gal. of fluids into the calf within a 24-hour period.

A Realistic Approach

No one vaccine nor any one type of antibiotic or chemotherapeutic agent will prevent calves from having scours. It is possible that certain bacteria over time develop resistance to antibiotics. A large percent of the microbial agents are resistant to most commonly-employed antibiotics. To assure that the proper antimicrobial agent is employed, antibiotic sensitivity should be determined by analyzing fecal cultures.

Vaccines can be produced successfully for one type of organism, but it is doubtful that vaccines can be produced for all of the infections which are thought to cause scours. A great deal is still to be learned about the nature of immunity to scours in the newborn calf.

More research is needed to answer this complicated problem. Tremendous changes in the calf's body are caused by scours. Dehydration, inflammation and electrolyte balance need to be considered in determining the proper treatment.

Rearing Calves From Several Origins

If you purchase dairy calves under 2 weeks of age from several different origins, here's how to get them off to a fast start:

☛ Place calves in individual stalls until 3 weeks old.

☛ Use a broad spectrum antibiotic administered intramuscularly.

☛ Administer an injection consisting of a combination of vitamins A, D and E.

☛ At first feeding, give a mixture of electroytes, glucose and 4 to 5 qts. water. For second, third and fourth feedings, give one-half of the usual amount of reconstituted milk replacer which is normally fed. After the fourth feeding increase the amount of milk replacer, following the recommendations of the milk replacer manufacturer, which is normally around 8% of the calf's weight. Maintain the water temperature used for diluting replacer at 100 degrees F.

☛ Keep fresh water in front of the calf at all times.

☛ Utensils used for feeding should be washed and sterilized after each feeding.

Chapter 36

Tips For Milking
Success In Your Herd

FOLLOWING THESE time-tested management practices can help you get more milk from your cows:

1 *Provide a good stress-free environment for your cows.*

If a cow becomes nervous or frightened, a hormone called adrenalin is released into the bloodstream. This blocks the effects of oxytocin—the hormone which stimulates milk let-down. This results in incomplete milking and consequently, reduced profits for you.

To prevent the release of adrenalin, cows should be treated gently and disturbances such as dogs barking should be kept to a minimum.

2 *Strip foremilk.*

Removal of the foremilk prior to washing the udder and teats is thought to significantly reduce the incidence of new infections. By doing this, the bacteria-laden foremilk is removed and is not forced up into the udder cistern by the washing process which could lead to new infections.

This management practice not only gives you an opportunity to check for abnormal milk and mastitis infections, but also provides additional stimulation for proper milk letdown.

3 *Wash and stimulate the cow's udder. Dry teats with individual paper towels.*

Cows must be properly prepared for efficient and healthy milking. The udder should be washed with warm (110 degrees F.) water containing a mild, non-irritating sanitizer. Washing the udder sends nerve impulses to the cow's brain and pituitary gland which then releases oxytocin.

Do not use excess water. If the udder is clipped and is clean, wash only the bottom of the udder and the teats. Predipping the washed teats with the proper teat is recommended.

Disposable paper towels should be used for washing and wiping the udder and shoud be thrown away after one use. This prevents bacteria and other microorganisms from being carried from one cow to the next. Even a clipped and clean-appearing udder may carry millions of bacteria. The udder and teats should be dried with a second paper towel immediately after washing to prevent gravitation of bacteria-laden water to the teat end. If predipping is done, be sure to thoroughly dry the teats with a paper towel.

4 *Apply the milking machine 45 seconds to 60 seconds after the start of stimulation.*

Milk letdown usually begins about 1 minute after washing and continues for 2 to 4 minutes. The optimal time for attaching the milker is 45 seconds to 60 seconds after washing.

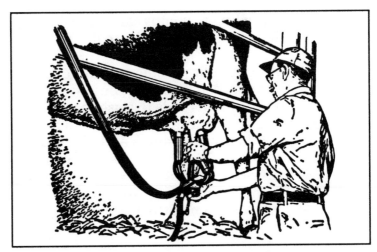

MILK LETDOWN. This usually starts about 1 minute after you wash the udder. The best time to attach the milker is normally 45 to 60 seconds after washing the cow's udder.

The milker unit operates on a system of differential pressures. The slightly higher udder pressure, coupled with the vacuum or reduced air pressure which occurs at the teat end, causes the milk to overcome the sealing action of the sphincter muscle. Milk then flows into the lower air pressure inside the machine, just as if you would let the air rush out of an inflated tire on your car or truck.

Pulsation alternates the low-pressure milking phase with the rest phase. The pulsator allows air to enter between the teat cup shell and the inflation which causes the inflation to collapse. The collapse creates a massaging effect, stimulating circulation in the teat walls.

5 *Adjust the milking machines for both downward and forward milking action.*

Be sure to properly adjust the milker unit to prevent the teat cups from crawling up on the teats.

Crawling teat cups can cause damage to the annular ring as well as the teat itself.

As the milk is removed, there is a tendency for a gradual collapse of the duct system. The collapse of this system tends to close the constriction between the teat and gland cistern. This lets the lateral sections of the ducts and gland sag, leaving up to 20% to 25% of the milk in the smaller ducts and alveoli. This trapped milk can most effectively be removed by using an alternating forward-downward motion of the teat cups.

6 *Avoid overmilking.*

When the udder is milked out, remove teat cups gently so as not to admit air.

Each teat cup should be removed separately. One or two quarters are usually "milked out" before the others. To remove cups individually, break the vacuum by pressing in on the teat with one finger just above the teat cup as the vacuum hose to the teat is crimped or pinched off. This can be done quite easily and quickly.

A carelessly removed inflation may allow enough air to flow into the milking unit to cause a large vacuum fluctuation and increase the possibility of backwashing bacteria-laden milk droplets to the other teats. This backwashing can be minimized by use of a four-chambered milking unit.

If individual inflations cannot be properly removed or when milking with claw-type units, the vacuum to the unit should be shut off prior to removal.

Teat cups should not be allowed to touch the floor because they will pick up dirt and bacteria. Keep-

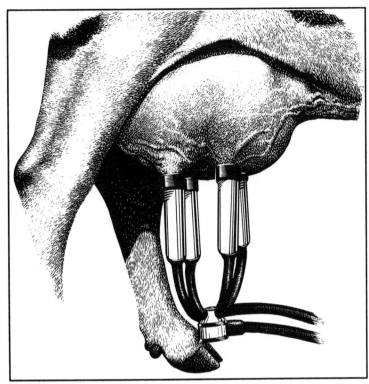

SELECT FOR FAST MILKING. Since hard or slow milking is a 20% to 35% heritable trait in dairy cattle, it will certainly pay you to select replacement heifers from cows and herd sires which are carrying valuable genetics for easy milking.

ing hair on the udder clipped short also helps prevent dirt from getting into the teat cups and makes washing the udder much quicker and easier.

The time required to milk will certainly vary, depending on breed and production capacity. It usually takes 3 to 6 minutes per cow. Some cows are hard or slow milkers. This trait is between 20% and 35% heritable—enough to make selection of replacements from cows and herd sires carrying the trait for easy milking worthwhile.

The individual doing the milking significantly affects required milking time, too. Operating too many units contributes to over-milking. Two or three units are considered the maximum per operator unless the operator is using automatic detachers. Whether two or three units are used should depend on other responsibilities during milking. Prolonged over-milking not only causes the cow to expect it, but also contributes to udder stress and injury. This may cause later slow milking problems.

7 *Dip the teats immediately after milking with an effective product.*

Research has shown spraying or dipping teats after each milking can reduce new infections by 50%.

To get the most out of dipping, the teat should be dipped two-thirds of the way up. If spraying is used, spray all the way around the teat. In either case, the bottom end of the teat should get a thorough cover to protect the teat sphincter. That's where organisms enter the mammary system. In addition, dipped teats are generally less likely to attract flies.

Chapter 37

Milking Management Score Card

HOW DOES YOUR your milking management really rate?

Give yourself three points for each question you can answer with a yes. A score of 99 or above indicates you are doing a good job on the most important management items to keep mastitis under control. A score of 69 or less may mean potential trouble. A low score may also indicate you are spending more time in the milking barn each day than is necessary.

Milking Procedures

Do You...

Stimulate the cow for milk letdown by washing and massaging the teats and udder for at least 25 to 30 seconds?

Attach the machine 1 minute after starting udder preparation?

Use individual paper towels to wash the udder?

Use a sanitizing solution in the wash water?

Use individual paper towels to dry the udders?

Machine strip your cows for not more than 15 seconds?

Turn off the source of vacuum and break the vacuum seal at the base of the teat before removing the machine?

Dip teats in an effective teat dip immediately after the teat cups are removed?

Avoid exciting the cows and try to handle them gently so they associate milking with a pleasant experience?

Follow a regular routine which your cows can expect at each milking?

Milk heifers and then cows with healthy udders first?

Milk mastitis-infected cows last?

Operate no more than two bucket-type milker units per man or not more than three units with a pipeline?

Milking Machines

Do You...

Have a milking machine representative check your equipment every 6 months?

Change rubber liners (inflations) every 1,200 cow milkings?

Clean your vacuum controllers as often as recommended by the manufacturer and local company which installed your milking system equipment?

Operate the machine at the vacuum level recommended by the manufacturer?

Keep milking equipment free of milk soils and protein buildup?

Clean and check pulsators at least once a month?

Clean the vacuum lines regularly?

Check for even, steady vacuum on the line and at the milker unit?

Wash equipment according to recommendations after each milking?

Prevention, Detection, Treatment

Do You...

Emphasize good management practices to prevent mastitis? (sanitizer in udder wash, individual towel, no over-milking, teat dip).

Raise your own replacements and buy no mature milking cows?

Raise calves in individual calf stalls until milk feeding is discontinued?

Breed cows with well-attached udders?

Sell cows with badly damaged udders?

Use a strip cup to detect mastitis and to further stimulate milk letdown?

Use California Mastitis Test paddles to detect mastitis?

Record the California Mastitis Test results, flare-ups and treatments used on each cow?

With DHIA testing, do you utilize the somatic cell count program?

Have a herd-health contract or mastitis control program with your veterinarian?

Call your veterinarian for help in prevention and treatment when mastitis increases in your herd?

Milking Time—Harvest Time!

Since your cows must be milked two or three times daily, milking may at times become monotonous. However, it must be done well—every time!

Remember that milking time is harvest time. The kind of job you do will be reflected in your level of milk production and returns you get from your herd. It will pay you well to do a good job.

Chapter 38

Keeping Score With Dairy Herd Health

USE THIS herd health scorecard to help you evaluate your present dairy management practices and comparative goals.

Mastitis Control/Quality Milk

The following management and health ideas can help you do a better job of producing top quality milk from your dairy herd.

Management Practices

Properly wash and dry all udders with individual towels.

Remove and properly examine foremilk.

Check all of your milking equipment at least twice annually.

Conduct premilking and postmilking teat dipping.

Use dry cow therapy for all cows.

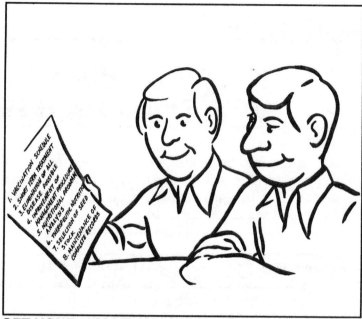

SET YOUR HEALTH GOALS. Just like with any type of management program, taking the time to set up the essential goals is a real key to your overall dairy health success.

Setting Disease Control Goals

The portion of the milking herd under health treatment at any given time—1% or less.

Herd somatic cell count—200,000 to 300,000.

California Mastitis Test Scores—85% or more negative.

Individual somatic cell count test—300,000 or less.

Standard plate count (raw count)—10,000 or less.

After pasteurization—100 or less.

Coliform count—10 or less.

Reproduction

To help you do a more efficient job of keeping your cows on the proper breeding and calving schedule, study these practices and goals closely.

Management Practices

Provide a separate calving area.

Schedule a regular veterinary examination of all cows before breeding.

Hold an annual review of heat detection and artificial insemination procedures.

Make early pregnancy diagnosis (35 to 65 days after breeding).

Use a veterinarian-designed vaccination program.

Goals For Reproduction

Calving interval—12 to 13 months.

Average days open per cow—50 to 75 days.

First service conceptions—60% or more of your cows.

Average services per conceptions—1.85 breedings or less.

Missed heats—15% or less of your cows.

Cows with retained placentas—5% of your cows or less.

Cows ready to breed (30 days postpartum)—95% or more of your cows.

Early embryonic death (before 50 days)—5% or less.

Abortion (after 50 days gestation)—3% or less of your cows.

Replacement Heifers

There is no easy way to properly select replacement heifers for your herd. But the following ideas may help you do a better job.

Management Practices

Provide a clean well bedded calving area away from the dairy herd.

Hand-feed quality colostrum milk before 6 to 12 hours of age.

Use individual calf pens.

Begin health records at birth.

Follow a professionally-formulated feeding program (birth through 24 months).

Follow a proper vaccination program.

Follow a successful parasite control program.

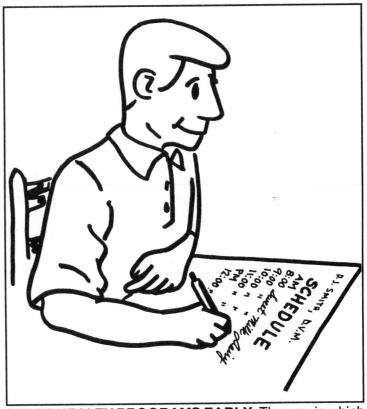

START HEALTH PROGRAMS EARLY. The way in which you manage and set goals for disease control in your heifer rearing program will have a big impact on profits you earn.

Disease Control Goals

Mortality to 8 weeks of age—5% or less of your calves.

Mortality and culling—3% or less of your animals.

Weaning—before 8 weeks.

Weight at calving (larger breeds)—1,300 lbs.

Age at calving—24 to 26 months.

General Herd Health

Carrying out a detailed dairy herd health management program can return big dividends for you for every dollar you spend on health care.

Management Practices

Have regularly scheduled veterinary visits.

Follow a complete herd vaccination program.

Use professional nutritional guidance.

Use a complete and current breeding and health record-keeping system.

Utilize DHIA testing.

Disease Control Goals

Cows culled for disease or injury—15% or less.

Total cows culled—35% or less.

Cows which die—3% or less.

Annual herd production level—figure on a 5% to 10% yearly increase.

Three Critical Keys

Remember that the success of any health program in your dairy herd depends on three key areas: prevention, detection and treatment.

Chapter 39

Using Your Sow And Litter Record Sheets

EFFECTIVE SWINE management certainly requires you to keep accurate and complete records on all of your sows and their litters. If you are to be successful in the hog business, there's no replacement for keeping proper breeding, production, veterinary and health records. These kinds of records will pay for themselves many times over!

Identifying Your Hogs

The first step in effectively using swine record cards, which are available from this book's publisher, is to properly identify your hogs with an ear notching system. The system we recommend for this purpose is explained in another chapter.

After ear notching has been done at an early age, it is easy to mark the identifying notches in the ear diagram in the upper right hand corner of the record sheet as well as to record the sow's number as shown by the ear-notching system.

The other information which is asked for on the top of the card is supplementary information which will prove most helpful in making all-important management decisions concerning your own hog operation.

Date Bred	Sire	Date Far-rowed	No. Born Dead	At Birth boars	At Birth Gilts	At 56 Days Boars	At 56 Days Gilts	At Birth	56 Days	When Sold	Litter Identifi-cation No.

Sow & Litter — Production, Breeding and Health Record

Sow's Name or No. _____

Registration No. _____ Breed _____

Her Dam _____ ( )Purebred ( )Grade ( )Crossbred

Her Sire _____ Source of Sow _____

NUMBER ALIVE / LITTER WEIGHT

Right / Left

FRONT OF SOW & LITTER CARD. This card has plenty of room for recording all the valuable breeding and production information for each of your sows and their offspring.

Breeding Records

Breeding records are an absolute requirement of any good swine management program. No successful hogman would ever attempt a breeding and farrowing program without keeping such records. However, too often such information is entrusted to memory or recorded in so many places that it isn't readily available when it is needed.

These sow and litter record cards have plenty of space for the date bred, the sire used and the date farrowed. Under normal circumstances this is all the breeding information you will need.

Production, Performance Records

Found immediately next to the breeding record part of the lined form is plenty of lined space for recording the necessary information on the members of the sow's litter.

The only way to judge the performance record of a sow is by the size of the litters she produces, by the conformation of the pigs in the litter at 56 days or at market age. In addition, some hogmen also like to record the weight of the litter at birth.

Wise breeders generally prefer to select breeding stock from litters that raised ten or more pigs. They want the pigs in the litter to reach market weight as soon as possible.

By ear-notching the pigs in the litter at birth and weighing them at 56 days or at market time, it is possible to select the best breeding animals for your herd. All of this information, including the litter identification number established by ear-notching, can be recorded in spaces provided on the number card.

Sow Name or No. _____

VETERINARY RECORD

Litter No	Date Farrowed	Date Castrated	Date Wormed	Date Other	Vaccination Record

HEALTH RECORD

Date	Symptom	Diagnosed As	Results

BACK SIDE OF SOW & LITTER CARD. This side of the card provides room for documenting all of the essential veterinary and health record info for each sow and her litter.

Veterinary, Health Records

On the back of the record card, you will find adequate space for a complete veterinary and health record of the sow and her litters. In the veterinary section (at the back side of the card) a record should be kept of the date farrowed, date castrated, date wormed and the vaccination record (date and for what disease).

The lower part of this same back page on the card provides a handy health record for the sow.

Try This Helpful Coding System

The B-2-4-6-8-10 rule is a helpful code that many producers have used over the years for success with hogs. This code makes it easier to remember the important things to do and when to do them in raising hogs:

B—Be there at farrowing time and clip needle teeth as well as ear-notch all baby pigs.

2—Castrate male pigs, give iron shots to all pigs and provide creep feed at 1 to 10 days of age.

4—Wean at 4 weeks.

6—Vaccinate at 6 weeks.

8—Deworm at 8 weeks.

10—Place pigs in grower pens at 10 weeks.

Good swine records are a must for successful swine management. By using these records for your sows and their litters, it will help you become a much better hogman.

Chapter 40

Properly Identifying Hogs For Record Keeping Purposes

TO MAKE money with hogs, you need big litters of lean-type pigs from your sows. To accomplish this, you must constantly select and cull your breeding stock.

But before you can select and cull properly, you need to know which sows and boars produce large litters and which large litters are bringing the highest market prices. You will know which sows and boars are the kind you want only if you have some method of positively identifying every animal in your herd. This is why identification of baby pigs is very important to you.

Proper Identification Is Necessary

The various kinds of records you should keep—which are all based on some form of positive animal identification—include sow production records, breeding and health records, plus pedigree and herd records.

How To Ear Notch

Since ear tags and similar markers are easily lost by swine, ear notching is usually used and recommended as a very effective means of identification by swine authorities and breeding associations. In fact, most swine breed associations require that pigs be ear-marked to be registered.

Ear-notching as soon as possible after farrowing is desirable. It helps prevent errors in putting pigs in the wrong litter and there is less bleeding when this is done very early in life. Breed associations also require that this be done at farrowing time to prevent costly litter mix-ups.

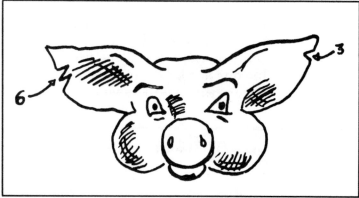

KEEP IT SIMPLE! Ear notch marking of pigs follows a simple code system. Reading the ear notches, this pig is number 63 which means he is from the sixth litter and the third pig marked in the litter. The pig's right ear has two marks which add up to six and tell you he is from the sixth litter.

The pig's left ear has a notch in the three zone to identify him with a number within the litter. On your record cards, you would identify him simply as number 63—knowing that the first numeral in the double number tells his litter while the last numeral provides his order in the particular litter.

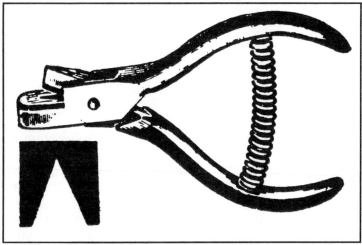

EAR MARKER. This is a typical and popular type of ear marker for identifying little pigs. Note the size and shape of the notch which it will cut in a little pig's ears. Smaller than most general purpose ear notchers, it is more convenient to handle and will enable you to make a smaller notch.

Ear notch marking of baby pigs is done with a small plier type tool especially made for this job. Its triangular blade cuts a small notch out of the fragile ear which normally heals quickly.

There is no need to clean or treat the ear if this ear notching is done when pigs are very young. If you want to treat ear notch wounds, use a good antiseptic or healing powder recommended for livestock. A good powder now on the market combines sulfa and urea and is believed to be especially effective.

When you notch, take a full triangular-shaped piece out of the ear so it will not grow shut. Depending on the size and age of the pig, this notch should be 3/8 to 1/2 in. deep.

Although numerous hog marking systems are used, we will explain here only the one adopted by most swine breed associations. This system has

individual Pig Notches

EAR NOTCHING SYSTEM. This system was designed to identify litters and pigs in litters. The right ear is used for the litter mark. All pigs in the same litter must have the same ear notches placed in this ear. Remember that the right ear is located on the pig's own right side. The left ear is used for notches to show an individual pig's own number in the litter. Every pig will have a different notch in this ear.

gained wide acceptance with swine producers because it provides positive identification with a minimum possibility of error.

It can be used to mark both the litter number and the pig number within the litter. Not all marking systems identify the individual pig. Instead they simply use one number for an entire litter or sow.

Give Each Pig A Number

Pigs in your litters can be numbered for your own records by placing a litter mark in the right ear and an individual pig mark in the left ear. Thus, a pig in the eighth litter whose individual number is nine becomes pig 89 on your records. When the litter number or individual pig number is two or more digits, an "X" can be placed after or before the number so they can be separated. For example, pig number nine in the fifty-first litter becomes pig 51X9 on the record card or the eleventh pig in the

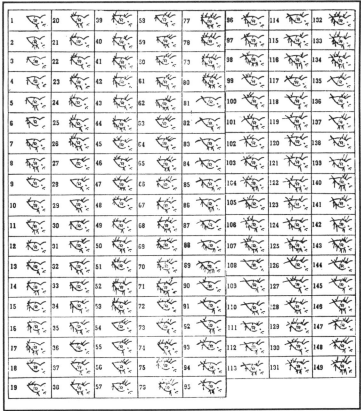

TAKE YOUR CHOICE. Each of these ear notches made in the pig's right ear identify the litter number. You can mark up to 149 litters with the notches shown here. Litter numbers and notches for the numbers are shown in each block.

eighth litter becomes pig No. 8X11. However, some swine producers prefer to use a dash instead of an X. But there is little difference as long as your system is uniform and you carefully follow it each time that you notch pigs.

Other Identification Methods

Other methods of identification are also used in addition to ear notching, but remember that the only official system of identification for registration with your breed association is the notching system they have accepted. However, swine owners who do not register purebred hogs may be interested in one of the following systems:

Ear Tags

There are many kinds of ear tags for hogs on the market. About 95% of the tags stay in, but some of them will pull out, making it almost impossible to identify the hog. As a result, accumulated records are often useless.

Ear tags for hogs are made of metal or plastic. Experience shows the plastic tags are easier to read and less apt to be lost. Different colored plastics can be the sole identification for different litters if there are not too many hogs on your farm.

Ear Rings

For the man with only a few hogs, the type of rings used for nose rings may be satisfactory to mark a few litters. Any system can be developed, but usually each ring stands for one. Thus, two rings in the pig's right ear, for example, stands for the second litter. A hog will occasionally pull one ring out but they seldom lose them all. If rings are lost, the holes left in the ear will usually help identify the animal.

Branding

Branding of hogs includes either chemical branding or hot iron branding.

In chemical branding, a commercial paste preparation of coal tar and sodium hydroxide is painted on. The chemical burns or "clips" off the hair. This chemical paste is put on where it's not likely to rub off before it leaves its mark. Any system can be used. For example, one group of gilts could have no mark, a second group could have a mark down the middle of the back and a third group could have a mark on one side.

While this branding system is more or less temporary, it gives some sort of identification which is helpful for breeding purposes, if not record keeping.

Branding with a hot iron is being used by more swine owners and seems to be more permanent than the chemical method. Remember that brand-

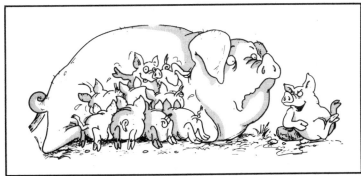

IDENTIFICATION RELIABILITY COUNTS. While several other means of identifying hogs are often used by producers, they are not as accurate or long-lasting as ear notching. Despite the extra work involved, most breed associations still demand ear notching of registered pigs.

ing hogs is trickier than branding cattle. One problem is getting the brand burned deep enough to show without getting it too deep and ending up with a festering sore that proves hard to heal.

For best results with hot iron branding, clip the hair from the area to be branded high on the side behind the shoulders. Burn the hogs deep with a 6-in. iron when they are selected as gilts. You must burn deep to inflict a first degree burn for good identification. Each time the sow farrows, clip the hair for easier identification of the brand.

Hogmen using this method report a hot brand will last through as many as eight farrowings. After the branded gilt farrows, you will usually find the brand can't be read easily when she leaves the farrowing house with her litter. But by the time the litter is weaned and the sow is ready for rebreeding, the brand can again be read easily. It can still be read at farrowing time if the hair is clipped.

Chapter 41

Managing Diseases In Your Swine Herd

USE THE INFORMATION found in this chapter to help you identify and treat those diseases which may affect your swine herd.

TGE

Stage of Growth: Baby pigs.

Prevention: Sow vaccination. Closed herd.

Treatment: Electrolytes. Milk replacer.

Drug Withdrawal Period: None.

Clostridial Enteritis

Stage of Growth: Baby pigs.

Prevention: Vaccination of sows with toxoid.

Treatment: Antitoxin at birth.

Drug Withdrawal Period: None.

Pseudorabies

Stage of Growth: All ages, including baby pigs.

Prevention: Vaccination. Select the type of vaccine which is recommended by your state veterinarian. Isolation of herd, quarantine and testing of herd replacements may also be needed.

Treatment: Vaccination in case of an outbreak may save some animals.

Drug Withdrawal Period: None.

Atrophic Rhinitis

Stage of Growth: Pigs older than 8 weeks.

Prevention: Vaccinate sows before farrowing. Vaccinate pigs at 7 to 21 days of age. Feed Chlortetracycline at 100 grams per ton, sulfathiazole at 100 grams per ton or penicillin at 50 grams per ton.

Treatment: Same as steps outlined for prevention of this disease.

Drug Withdrawal Period: 15 days.

Pneumonia

Stage of Growth: All ages.

Prevention: Prevent drafts. Avoid chilling of pigs.

Treatment: Oxytetracycline, Penicillin, Tylosin, Lincomycin or Tiamulin.

Drug Withdrawal Period: It will range from 2 to 36 days, depending on the drug and particular formulation used. Check the drug label.

Anemia

Stage of Growth: Baby pigs.

Prevention: Provide injectable iron at 1 to 3 days of age. Give only 100 mg.

Treatment: Same as outlined under prevention.

Drug Withdrawal Period: None.

Colibacillosis (E. Coli)

Stage of Growth: Baby pigs up to 5 weeks of age.

Prevention: Feed bacterin to sow 5 and 3 weeks before farrowing. Strict sanitation. Avoid chilling.

Treatment: Nitrofurazone or Gentamycin in drinking water for 3 days.

Drug Withdrawal Period: 5 to 10 days.

Leptospirosis

Stage of Growth: All ages.

Prevention: Vaccinate all breeding animals annually.

Treatment: Feed Oxytetracycline at a recommended rate of 500 grams per ton of feed.

Drug Withdrawal Period: 5 days.

Parvovirus

Stage of Growth: Gilts and sows. Boars can also shed this virus.

Prevention: Vaccinate animals. Allow gilts and sows to co-mingle.

Treatment: None.

Erysipelas

Stage of Growth: Animals of all ages.

Prevention: Vaccinate sows prior to breeding and then again 5 weeks after breeding. Vaccinate pigs at 6 to 8 weeks of age.

Treatment: Penicillin (injectable) anti swine or E serum.

Drug Withdrawal Period: 5 days.

Mycoplasma Ssp

Stage of Growth: Growing and finishing swine. Older animals may also be carriers.

Prevention: Vaccinate pigs at weaning time. Repopulate only with clean breeding animals.

Treatment: Lincomycin, Tiamulin or Oxytetracycline fed according to recomendations.

Drug Withdrawal Period: It should be 1 to 6 days depending on the drug and particular formulation used. Check the drug label carefully.

Swine Dysentery

Stage of Growth: Affects pigs from 40 lbs. to market age.

Prevention: Isolate all new animals. Feed arsanilic acid at 90 grams per ton of feed. Add 50 to 200 grams per ton of BMD to feed.

Treatment: Tiamulan, Carbadox (up to 75 lbs.) or BMD at 200 grams per ton.

Drug Withdrawal: It will range from 3 to 70 days with these products. Check the drug label.

Haemophilus Pleuro-Pneumonia

Stage of Growth: Affects pigs of all ages.

Prevention: Vaccination.

Treatment: Individual treatment consists of Penicillin injectable or Oxytetracycline. For herd treatment, use Tiamulin.

Drug Withdrawal Period: It ranges from 3 to 26 days for these drugs and available formulations. Check drug label carefully.

Jowl Abscesses

Stage of Growth: Finishing pigs.

Prevention: Chlortetracycline at 50 to 100 grams per ton.

Treatment: Penicillin (injectable).

Drug Withdrawal Period: 5 days.

Parakeratosis

Stage of Growth: 20 to 50 lb. pigs.

Prevention: Add 50 parts per million of zinc to the ration.

Treatment: Add 50 parts per million of zinc to the ration.

Drug Withdrawal Period: None.

Edema Disease

Stage of Growth: 20 to 40 lb. pigs.

Prevention: Avoid sudden changes in the environment.

Treatment: Add Nitrofurazones to drinking water.

Drug Withdrawal Period: 5 days.

Internal Parasites

Stage of Growth: All ages.

Prevention: Worm sows prior to farrowing. Worm pigs at 40 lbs.

Treatment: Use Fenbendazole or a Ivermectin injection. Talk with your veterinarian regarding the best parasite treatment products for you to use in order to effectively control the particular internal parasite problems that may be present in your swine herd.

Drug Withdrawal Period: 3 days to 18 days for these products. Read the label.

External Parasites

Stage of Growth: Pigs of all ages, including the breeding herd.

Prevention: Use Lindane, Prolate, Permethrin, Tactic or an Ivermectin injection.

Treatment: You can use the same program as for prevention.

Drug Withdrawal Period: Read the label carefully, as these products have withdrawal periods that range from 1 to 30 days.

Chapter 42

Swine Schedule To Use With Your Farrow-To-Finish Program

BY FOLLOWING this recommended and time-tested management and health program, you can keep your swine herd operating at peak capacity and earn top profits.

Prebreeding

Carry out the following program 2 to 4 weeks prior to breeding your gilts or sows:

Vaccinate for Leptospirosis (5 way).

Vaccinate for erysipelas.

Vaccinate for parvovirus (especially gilts).

Deworm gilts and sows with Safeguard.

Allow gilts to co-mingle with sows 3 weeks prior to breeding.

Place boars in close proximity to gilts and weaned sows.

Increase the energy intake (flushing during breeding period) for gilts and sows. Resume the feeding of your normal sow or gilt ration just as soon as is possible after the breeding is finished.

Allow more than one breeding during each heat period—but use a different boar for the second breeding.

Gestation

Vaccinate for Clostridium perfringens, TGE, Erysipelas and E. coli 3 to 4 weeks prior to farrowing.

Don't administer all vaccines at the same time.

Deworm sows 1 week prior to farrowing.

Spray for lice and mange at the same time.

Wash sows immediately prior to placing them in the farrowing area.

Start feeding a lactation ration 1 week prior to farrowing.

Farrowing, Lactation

Newborn pig area should be kept at 90 to 95 degrees F.—the sow area should be 65 degrees F.

Farrowing stalls should be steam cleaned. If possible, steam clean again in 3 days.

Continue feeding your sow lactation ration for 3 days after birth.

Slowly start to increase the amount of feed to the sow so she will be on full feed in 7 days.

Clip needle teeth—don't break them off and leave splinters.

Give iron (150 mg) on second day after farrowing.

Reduce heat for pigs to 65-70 degrees F.

Vaccinate pigs for atrophic rhinitis, erysipelas nd mycoplasma at 7 to 10 days of age. Repeat again in 10 days.

Castrate pigs at 1 to 10 days of age.

Wean pigs at 21 to 25 days of age.

Grower (Nursery)

Deworm at 8 weeks if pigs have not been placed on wire mesh floors.

Spray for lice and mange.

Vaccinate for pseudorabies 2 weeks after weaning if you are located in a problem area.

Rebreeding Sows

Sows should be kept in close proximity to boars 1 week after farrowing.

Limit feed to 6 to 8 lbs. per sow after weaning.

Double mate during heat period. Provide one boar for every five sows.

Reduce each sow's feed to 4 to 5 lbs. after breeding.

Pregnancy check sows 35 to 40 days after breeding.

Sell all females that are not pregnant.

Finishing

Observe all swine daily.

Immediately isolate sick, depressed or scouring animals.

Deworm and spray for lice and mange if it is has been 30 days since the last dewormer was used.

Use a growth promotant.

Note: The use of vaccines for Hemophilus pleuro-pneumonia and pseudorabies should be used only after consultation with your veterinarian.

Chapter 43

How To Clip Those Baby Pig Needle Teeth

AT BIRTH, baby pigs have four long, sharp teeth on each jaw. These sharp teeth, found in the forward part of the mouth, are usually black or brown in color, while a pig's other teeth are white.

These are commonly called needle or wolf teeth. Longer and sharper than other teeth in the pig's mouth, they can cause considerable trouble in a litter of baby pigs.

Pig needle teeth often cut into and irritate the sow's udder as the pig nurses, causing infection and injury. As a result, a sow may refuse to nurse pigs, limiting their food supply and causing runts or even death.

Long needle teeth are really small tusks. If allowed to remain in the pig's mouth, they can also result in pigs injuring one another. These long teeth or fangs are vestiges of the early wild boar. Pigs will naturally use them to fight unless they are removed. When fighting, pigs with needle teeth can inflict wounds that cause disease infections. Wounds about the head can cause severe infections.

Clip Teeth Early

Baby pig needle teeth should be removed right after birth. If pigs injure the sow at their first attempt to suckle, the new mothers—especially gilts—may refuse to let the entire litter nurse. Sows become nervous and may kill or injure pigs even though they allow nursing. If needle teeth are allowed to remain, they may lacerate the sow's teats, causing the teats to become sore and preventing a sow from allowing the pigs to nurse properly.

Some hog producers mistakenly do not clip needle teeth because they believe the mouth and gums may be injured, allowing infectious organisms to enter the body. However, this mistaken impression was probably made by someone who performed this simple operation without proper care or instruction, leaving sharp stubs of teeth or bruising and cutting the pig's gums. If done properly, clipping baby pig needle teeth will not cause infections and can actually help prevent them.

Preparing For The Job

Some hog producers remove needle teeth and also ear notch baby pigs at the same time. See another chapter of this book for ear notching suggestions and instructions.

Be sure you use the correct type of teeth nippers or pliers. They should be designed so the sharp cutting edges give a smooth clean break. Never use pliers which leave a broken, jagged edge that can sometimes be sharper than the needle teeth themselves and are apt to bruise or cut the gums. The ends of the cutting blades or nose of the pliers should be rounded and dulled, so you will not inadvertently punch or cut the gums or mouth of the pigs.

For the same reason, the nose of the pliers or the cutting blades should not be too long.

Diagonal cut wire pliers have been used for clipping pig teeth for many years. However, needle teeth cutters are available which are slightly smaller than most wire pliers, chrome plated to aid sanitation and equipped with a self-opening spring to facilitate one-handed use. Most importantly, these pig teeth nippers are especially designed with relatively short, blunt cutting edges to avoid the possibility of cutting the pig's mouth and causing infection.

Before starting, make sure the teeth nippers are clean by scrubbing them in a solution of alcohol. If alcohol is not available, a good scrubbing in hot soapy water will do the job. Soap and water is a satisfactory disinfectant if a liberal scrubbing is given.

Catching, Holding Pigs

Before catching pigs, separate the sow from the litter and pen her out of reach of both you and the pigs. While small pigs can be easily caught by hand, never hold pigs by the nose or tail. This causes them to scream and struggle, unnecessarily exciting the sow and making other pigs in the same litter more difficult to manage.

Small pigs are best caught by seizing one or both hind legs and swinging or lifting them from the floor. At the same time, shift your hands, so one supports the pig's belly just behind the front legs and the other presses down across the shoulders.

In this manner, a pig can be placed with the rump under your left arm and held tightly against your body with your elbow, freeing the left hand enough so you can grasp and hold the pig's head and shoulders with the left hand. Use the fingers of this same left hand to hold the pig's mouth open and expose the needle teeth. With the right hand, operate the teeth nippers.

Pig needle teeth are sharp enough to injure your fingers and hands, so use plenty of caution when placing fingers in a little pig's mouth.

Completing The Job

There are four needle teeth on both the bottom and top jaws of the pig, four on each side of the mouth. With the pig held in a way to make the teeth easily accessible, clip the needle teeth level with the other teeth. Do not try to cut the teeth level with the gums. Clipping at the level of the other teeth helps in avoiding damage to the pig's mouth.

Clip the teeth so you get a clean, smooth break with no jagged edges and no injury to the gums. Hold the nippers carefully and do not let the pig jerk to cut or bruise himself.

There is little need for treatment of the teeth and gums after nipping, providing ordinary sanitary precautions are taken. However, some hogmen prefer to place a drop or two of tincture of iodine on the teeth as an added precaution against infection.

Chapter 44

Castrating Your Pigs

THE CASTRATING of pigs can be easily done by the farmer himself, providing a number of proven techniques are followed carefully.

For best results and less set-back to the animals, castration should be performed when pigs are 1 to 10 days of age.

Choosing Castrating Equipment

Your choice of the proper castrating knife is very important. It must be sharp to do a fast and sanitary, but safe job. The old fashioned castrating knife is no longer popular for castrating small pigs. Although it is dangerous many farmers will use an open razor blade. Others use an expensive scalpel. The most satisfactory instrument is probably a razor blade knife. It uses a sharp, but easily replaced low cost razor blade. The protected blade

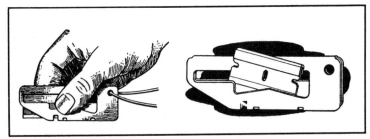

PRACTICAL CUTTING. This pig castrating knife uses a razor blade for the cutting edge. Dull blades are very easy to remove and can be replaced with a super-sharp blade.

slides in and out of its holder to limit the specific depth of cut. As an extra convenience, you can hang the knife from a string around your neck to free both hands to help catch and hold pigs.

Several good disinfecting powders and liquid solutions suitable for use on castration wounds are available. One recommended, low cost powder is a combination of sulfa and urea powder. It is quickly sprayed or puffed on from a plastic, squeeze bottle without touching the wound.

Two Castrating Methods To Use

There are two basic methods used in castrating swine. Use the one that seems to suit you best.

Method Number One

☛ Have a helper hold the pig belly up, with the animal's hind legs pulled forward and pressed into the belly.

☛ Clean and disinfect the scrotum and surrounding area with a good disinfecting material. This is very important.

☛ Massage one testicle into the bottom part of the scrotal sac and grasp it firmly between your forefinger and thumb. Stretch the skin tight at the point of incision, about 3/4 in. off the midline.

☛ Make an incision with a single bold stroke of your knife or blade through the baby pig's skin and into the meaty part of the testicle. This incision should be 1 1/2 to 2 in. long at the lower end of the

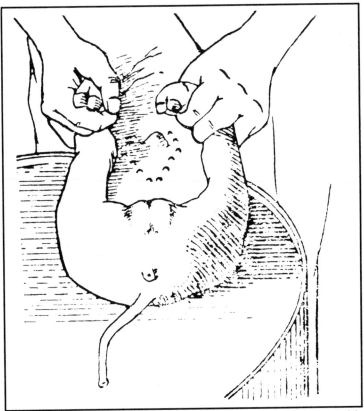

BELLY UP. Have a worker hold the baby pig belly up with hind legs pulled forward and pressed into the pig's belly.

scrotal sac to allow adequate drainage of the cut.

☞ Force the testicle through the incision by applying pressure with your thumb and forefinger. The membrane attached to the end of the testicle can be severed with the castrating instrument.

☞ Make the cord tight by pulling on the testicle. This will allow the whitish membranes to return to the scrotal sac. The sperm cord can then be pulled out with a quick jerk or by scraping it with the edge of a sharp knife.

313

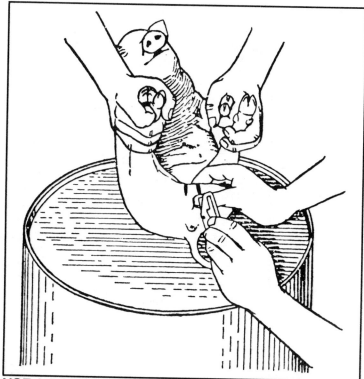

USE A BOLD KNIFE STROKE. Make an incision through the pig's skin and into the meaty part of the testicle. This cut should be 2 inches long at lower end of the scrotal sac.

☛ Repeat this same procedure through a second incision made in the same manner for the other testicle.

☛ During fly season, apply a fly repellent to the skin surface around the incision. Don't be in such a hurry as to avoid this step.

☛ Keep castrated pigs in clean and dry quarters for 24 to 48 hours. Never allow freshly castrated pigs into water holes, wallows or other places filled with excess moisture as infection can result.

Method Number Two

☞ Have a helper hold the pig by the rear legs, with its head down and belly out.

☞ Cleanse and disinfect the area carefully and thoroughly between the hind legs of the pig with a good disinfectant material. Again, this is very important in order to avoid costly infections at a later date.

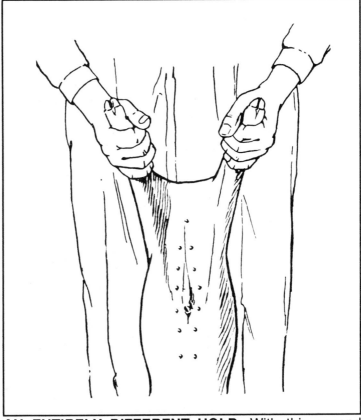

AN ENTIRELY DIFFERENT HOLD. With this second method of castration, have one of your helpers hold the pig by the rear legs, head down and with the belly pointing out.

☞ Locate and massage both testicles in a direction toward the pig's head until they are positioned between the rear legs.

☞ While continuing to apply downward pressure, make an incision directly over and into the testicle at least 1 1/2 to 2 1/4 in. long to allow easy removal and proper drainage.

☞ By applying pressure between your thumb and forefinger, force the testicle through the incision.

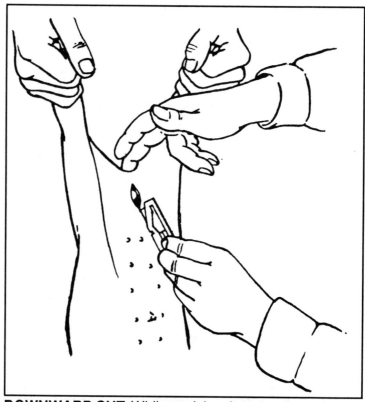

DOWNWARD CUT. While applying downward pressure to the pig's body, make a nearly 2 1/4 inch incision directly over and into the testicle. This will allow for easy removal.

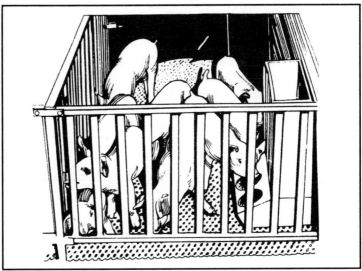

KEEP YOUR PIGS DRY AND CLEAN. Separate all newly-castrated pigs from other animals for 1 to 2 days. Keep them comfortable and check for possible infections.

☞ Holding the cord taut, slip the membranes back into the cavity and sever the cord as near the body as possible.

☞ Repeat the same procedure through a second

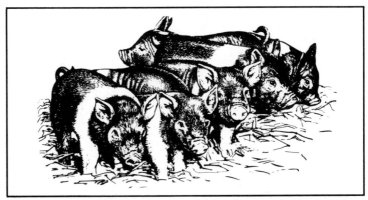

BEST RESULTS. For less costly setbacks for baby pigs, it is best to castrate when they are only a few weeks old.

incision made over the other testicle.

☞ During the fly season, be sure to apply a fly repellent to the skin surface around the incision. Do not omit this step.

☞ Keep the pigs in dry and clean quarters for 24 to 48 hours. Keep freshly castrated pigs away from water holes, wallows or other places with excess moisture to avoid health problems.

Chapter 45

Giving Shots To Your Hogs

BEFORE MAKING any kind of injection in your hogs, read the label on the bottle carefully. Be sure you fully understand all cautions, proper dosage, frequency of administration and recommended method of administration. In this chapter, we will provide you with detailed injection instructions.

Making An Intramuscular Injection

An intramuscular injection is made through the skin and subcutaneous tissue, directly into the muscle. Absorption is very rapid. It is commonly used in swine, cattle and sheep

Needed Equipment

- A 25 or 50-cc veterinary syringe.

- A hypodermic needle, 16 gauge, 3/4 to 1 in. in length.

- Scissors or clippers.

- 70% rubbing alcohol compound or other equally effective antiseptic for disinfecting the skin and bottle stopper.

- The medication to be given.

Preparing Your Equipment

Clean and disinfect the needles and syringe by boiling them in water for 20 minutes.

Areas Of Injection

An intramuscular injection is made directly into the muscle tissue or meat. Heavily muscled portions of the body such as the neck and shoulder should be utilized. Not more than 25-cc should be injected in any one spot in large animals such as heavy boars. In smaller pigs, not more than 10 to 15 cc of medicine should be injected in any one spot. Where the dosage to be given is large, it should be distributed in 25-cc amounts into the heavy muscles of the neck and shoulder on both sides of the animal.

Preparing The Animals

Restrain the animal by the best means available. Clip the hair from the area where the injection is to be given. Swab the clipped area vigorously with alcohol or another equally effective antiseptic solution.

Inserting The Needle

Fill the syringe with the medication to be given, using a separate needle for filling. Disinfect the rubber stopper before inserting the needle into the bottle.

Insert a previously disinfected needle deeply into the muscle tissue with a quick thrust. Observe the hub of the needle for a moment before going any further.

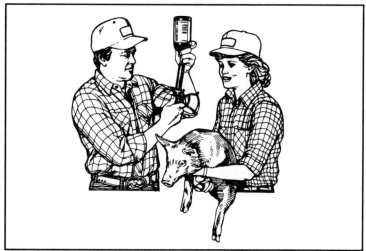

DO IT RIGHT! Giving shots to hogs is not all that difficult, However, make sure you make all injections properly so the drugs and other medicines can effectively do their job.

If blood begins to flow out of the needle, it is probably located in a blood vessel and the needle should be withdrawn and reinserted in a different direction. Attach the syringe to the needle and inject the medication slowly.

After the medication has been injected, remove the needle still attached to the syringe and massage the area with cotton soaked in alcohol to spread the medication through the muscle tissue. This procedure should be repeated in each injection area until the full recommended dose of medication has been given.

Making A Subcutaneous Injection

A subcutaneous injection is made directly into the body tissue beneath the skin.

As with an intramuscular injection, this type of

shot is also commonly used with swine, cattle and sheep.

First, read the directions again for making an intramuscular injection. The equipment needed, its preparation and preparation of the animal are the same as for making an intramuscular injection.

A subcutaneous injection is an injection made beneath the skin, such as between the skin and the muscle tissue. Recommended areas of injection are places where the skin is loose, particularly on the sides of the neck and behind the shoulder.

In pigs, the axillary space is frequently used for subcutaneous injections. The axillary space lies between the foreleg and the chest wall. It corresponds to the armpit on a man.

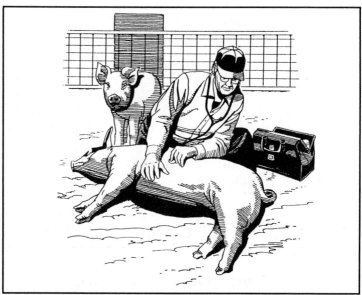

KNOW THE DIFFERENCES. Make sure you and all of your farm workers know the differences between the two types of injections. Each type serves a particular purpose.

To make the injection, pinch up a fold of skin between the thumb and fingers (this is not necessary if the axillary space is used). Insert the needle under the fold in a direction approximately parallel to the surface of the body.

When the needle is inserted in this manner, the medication will be delivered underneath the skin between the skin and the muscles. Observe the same precautions regarding clipping and disinfecting the skin as outlined under intramuscular injections.

Other Methods Of Administering Drugs

Several other methods of administering drugs to swine include the following:

Inhalation

(Inhale). Volatile drugs are used mainly because of their satisfactory local action on the respiratory tract.

Rectal

By the rectum. This method is used when oral administration is inadvisable or impossible because of paralysis of the throat, etc. Absorption of medication with this method is normally much slower than by injection.

Topical

Local application to external surfaces of the body. Absorption by this method is extremely slow and the effects of the drug are limited strictly to the treated area.

Oral

By the mouth. Drugs are usually given by mouth and are absorbed in the stomach and intestines. Absorption is more rapid when drugs are given in a solution into an empty stomach. Absorption is much slower when administered in powder, pill or ball form or into a full stomach.

Chapter 46

Effectively Moving And Handling Your Pigs

MANY VETERINARY and management practices require a swine producer to move or hold pigs. Although these procedures are normally relatively simple, they should be done correctly.

Moving, Loading Pigs

Bad handling and loading of pigs causes lost hours, bad tempers and bruised carcasses which are very costly to the swine industry. The single biggest loss in shipping hogs is shrink. Experts claim the largest losses due to shrink occur in the first 25% of the distance to be traveled and are caused almost entirely by fear and excitement. Handle pigs quietly and carefully.

Here's how to solve your handling problems and make your swine operation much more efficient:

If you cannot load your pigs directly from the finishing pens, drive them into the truck from a narrow passage, such as the alleyway in your finishing house.

Back the truck or trailer as close to the doorway as possible. Drop the loading chute and cover the side rails with sacks or other materials if possible. When pigs cannot see another way out, they are less likely to try to break away.

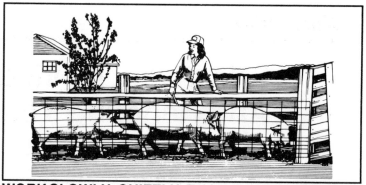

WORK SLOWLY, QUIETLY. Taking your time when loading pigs of any age will make the job much easier and result in less stress and injury for both your workers and animals.

Put plenty of straw or sand on the loading chute floor and in front of the ramp to prevent slipping and panic. Be sure the chute is not too steep, since pigs will load much easier up a gradual slope.

Drive pigs quietly and slowly. Walk behind them with a solid hurdle. Never use a cane or club to drive pigs because both cause bruises, frighten and excite the animals.

An electric prod powered by flashlight batteries is also a safe tool to use in loading pigs. When pigs become fearful and stubborn, scattering manure from their own pen over the loading chute and in the truck may help overcome strange smells. As a result, they will often load much easier.

Another loading method for use with a problem hog is to back it into the truck or trailer. A bucket placed over the head or a solid hurdle in front of the animals may do the trick. Remember that pigs will always try to back out of the way of something they cannot see through.

Boars can often be enticed into a truck by a sow. Sometimes you can also starve them a little before loading and encourage them to enter the vehicle with feed.

Breeding pigs need special care when loading. Treat them very gently, put plenty of straw or sand down and separate bred sows from other animals to avoid fighting.

Since hogs are highly susceptible to pneumonia, breeding stock should be transported in closed trucks during cold winter weather. Enough ventilation should be provided to prevent steaming and dampness problems.

Remember that a stick will only frighten pigs, cause bruises and damage to the carcass. Hog producers who handle and move large numbers of swine each year will find investing in a special loading ramp is a valuable asset.

Catching, Holding Pigs

For clipping teeth, earnotching, castrating, taking rectal temperatures and other veterinary and managerial practices, it is important to know how to catch and hold pigs correctly.

Never hold your pigs by the nose or tail as this causes them to scream, and struggle. It also makes their mates excited, fearful and much more difficult to manage.

Smaller-sized pigs that need to be caught for earnotching and other types of health work are best handled by seizing one or both of the hind legs and then swinging the animal clear of the floor.

At the same time, shift your hands so one hand

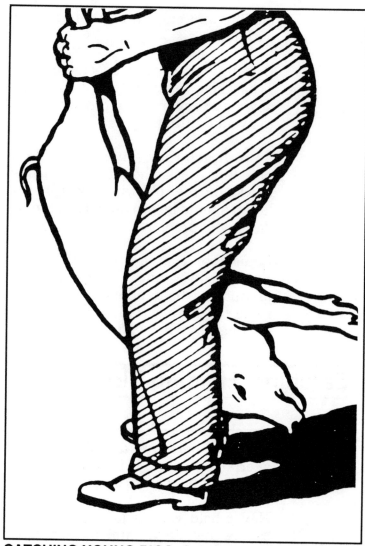

CATCHING YOUNG PIGS. Seize the pig by one or both hind legs and then easily swing the hog clear of the floor.

supports the pig's belly just behind the front legs while the other hand presses down across the animal's shoulders.

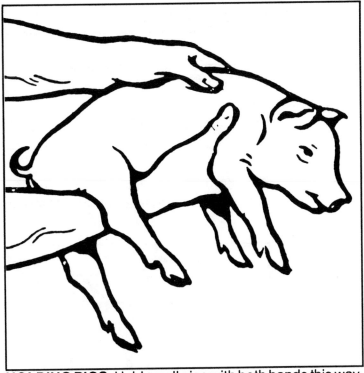

HOLDING PIGS. Hold small pigs with both hands this way.

Holding Weanling Pigs

These animals can be grasped by the hind legs and held head down in one of two different positions:

☛ Turn the pig's back towards you and squeeze its sides firmly between your knees.

☛ Turn the belly towards you and straddle the pig so your legs hold the animal in a scissors-like grip just behind the front quarters.

Holding Larger Pigs

These animals can be grasped by the front legs and held head up in one or two different positions:

☞ Set the pig on its haunches, belly facing away from you and clamp your knees against its ribs.

☞ Follow the same directions, but let the pig stand on its hind legs instead of sitting on its rump.

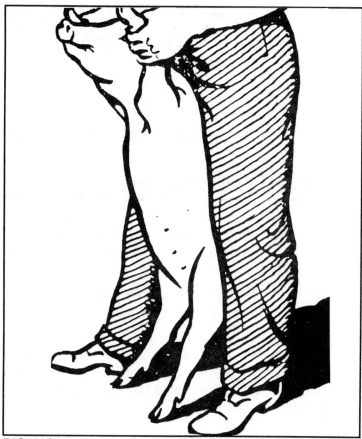

PIG HOLD. To properly and effectively hold a young animal, squeeze the pig's sides firmly between your knees.

Pigs which are not excessively large can also be held after being cast onto their backs by facing the head toward you. Grasp the two legs on the left side in the left hand and the other two legs in the right hand. The pig can then be held firmly by pressure that raises the hind quarters while the shoulders are forced down against the floor or table top.

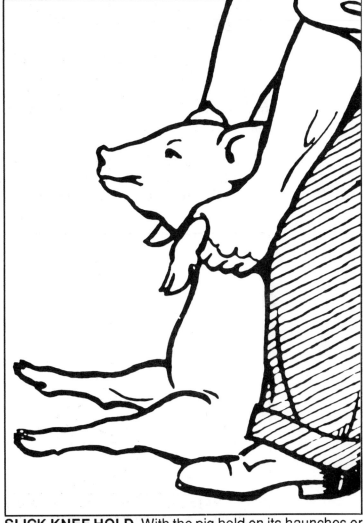

SLICK KNEE HOLD. With the pig held on its haunches or rump, clamp your knees against its ribs for a secure hold.

Holding Boars, Sows

Big boars and sows can often prove quite dangerous to handle. Such animals are best held by rope trusses or by "pig paralyzers."

All sizes of pigs can be kept completely under control with this device. To control the pig, the loop formed by the steel cable is slipped well back over the upper jaw and pulled tight.

Make sure you carefully wash your hands with hot soap and water after handling pigs with your bare hands. Pigs can transmit several diseases to humans. Avoid handling pigs if you have cuts or open sores on your hands.

Always wear leather gloves when handling larger pigs. Remember that a pig's bite is highly infectious; if bitten, see a doctor immediately.

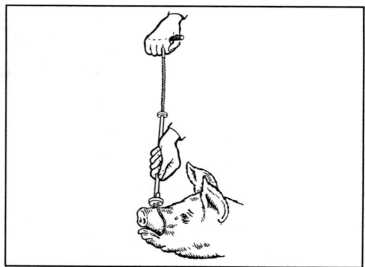

PIG PARALYZERS. To control the large boar or sow, the loop formed by the nylon covered steel cable is slipped well back over the upper jaw and pulled tight. Be careful with it.

Chapter 47

Using Your Ewe Record Sheets

TO MAKE MONEY with sheep and improve your flock, it is essential that you keep accurate, reasonably complete production records.

While the trained observer can effectively judge sheep breeding stock, only good records will show you the ability of particular rams and ewes to transmit growth rate, fleece quality and desirable conformation to their offspring. This information is needed to cull poor producers and build up your flock.

What Your Records Should Include

Your records should identify offspring and their parents. Birthdate, sex and final disposal of the lamb should also be recorded. Since the important factors in selecting breeding flock replacements and culling poor producers are growth rates, fleece weight, quality and prolificacy, these points along with desirable conformation should be determined and listed on your record card.

The Ewe Record Cards shown in this chapter provide you with a compact, permanent record of each ewe's production, health and veterinary services.

Properly Identify Ewes, Rams

The first necessary step to good sheep record keeping is to establish a method of permanently identifying ewes and rams. For this purpose, numbered ear tags have proven to be the best method.

Start a Ewe Record Card for each individual ewe in your flock. Fill in the card with as much information as you have available. If some information is lacking, make it your goal to gather these useful facts on future ewes. Your Ewe Record Cards can help you accumulate this information if properly kept up-to-date.

One item on the cards may need explanation. The abbreviations S, Tw, and Tr stand for single birth, twin or triplet.

Information On Ewe's Progeny

You may find it more practical to record the basic information in a note book. Then transfer it later to your permanent Ewe Record Cards, which provide space for essential breeding, lambing and production information.

As soon as the lamb is identified with an ear tag number, the number should be recorded on the card and the production record of that lamb jotted down on the right side of the card. Notice that the line for each year is split to allow you to record information for twins. Triplets, however, will require you to use an additional line.

While recording birth weight is not absolutely essential for managing your flock, it does provide valuable production information at an early age. It

| EWE | Production, Breeding and Health Record | | | | | | | | | | | | | | |

Ewe No. _____ Birth Date _____ S( )TW( )Tr( )

Reg. No. _____ Birth Weight (lbs.) _____ Sire No. & Breed _____

Breed(s) _____ Weaning Weight (lbs.) _____ Dam No. & Breed _____

Information on Ewe's Progeny

*Lamb Index: See reverse side for instructions

| | | Bred | | Date | Lamb | | Birth | | Weaning | | Fleece | | Lamb* | Disposal |
Year	Ram	Date	Date	Lambed	No.	Sex	Wt.	Grade	Wt.	Grade	Wt.	Grade	Index	Of Lambs

FRONT SIDE OF EWE CARD. Detailed information on the animal itself and breeding data, along with many different types of valuable records on its offspring, can be tabulated.

will be needed in determining a number of other important computations.

Weaning weight is very important. Since it is usually impractical to weigh lambs at exactly the same age, a commonly used method is to weigh all lambs about 120 days after the middle of your lambing period. The weight of each lamb should be recorded and then adjusted or corrected to a 120 day weight.

This can be done by subtracting birth weight from final weight and dividing this figure by the number of days of age of the lamb to get the average daily gain. By multiplying this figure by 120 and adding the birth weight, you will get an adjusted 120 day weight for each lamb.

☛ A simple formula for determining average daily gain would be:

Weaning weight minus birth weight divided by age

(in days) equals average daily gain.

☛ For determining the adjusted weight, the formula would be:

The lamb's average daily gain times 120 plus the actual birthweight in pounds equals the 120 day adjusted weight.

Grades (choice, good, utility) at birth and at weaning time, as well as the fleece grade, aren't always available. However, they will add information which is useful in indexing your flock. Many sheepmen with a minimum amount of experience determine these grades themselves for this record. Such information is very valuable if done uniformly.

Determining The Ewe Index

An ewe index based on production (see the left side of the back of your record card) is a valuable tool in selecting breeding stock and for culling. The index-

---

Ewe Index Points

Production Factor	Points
Single born, single raised	0
Twins born, single raised	5
Twins born, twins raised	10
Pounds of lamb per ewe, adjusted to 120 days	(Actual number lbs.)
Choice lamb grade	10
Good lamb grade	5
Utility Lamb grade	1
Wool, per pound	3

Ewe Index Based On Production				
Year	Lb Of Wool	No. Lambs Raised	Total Sale Wt. of Lambs	Ewe* Index

Ewe Health Record			
Date	Symptom	Diagnosed As	Results

How to figure Ewe or Lamb Index
Assign points as shown, then total

EWE		LAMB	
Production Factor	Pts.	Production Factor	Pts.
Single born, raised	0	3 times wool staple length in centimeters	
Twins born, single raised	5	Weight of Lamb (adjusted to 120 days	
Twins born, twins raised	10	Born as a twin, raised as a single	7
Pounds lamb per ewe (adjusted to 120 days)		Born as a twin, raised as a twin	14
Choice lamb	10		
Good lamb	5		
Utility lamb	1		
Wool (Pounds x 3)			
Total Record in Index		Total Record in Index	

Veterinary Record			
Date	Treatment Or Practice	For	Results

BACK SIDE OF EWE CARD. This sheet provides information for determing the ewe index along with recording plenty of essential health or veterinary record information.

ing system permits a very simple number comparison of one ewe's production with all other ewes in your flock.

While a number of different indexing systems are used, a system suggested some years back for sheepmen in Minnesota has proven to be simple and as accurate as most. This system gives a point value for each factor and these points are added together to obtain the ewe index. The key factors and their point values are shown in the table at left.

As an example as to how this index works, lets say an ewe has twins, but one dies shortly after birth. The remaining lamb has a 120 day adjusted weight of 80 lbs. and grades Good. Some 9 lbs. of wool are sheared. This ewe would then have a production index of 117 points (5 points of single raised of twin birth plus 80 lbs. plus 5 points for Good Choice plus 27 (9 lbs. of wool times 3) points equals 117 points).

After the ewe's index is calculated, it is recorded with other information on the back of the Ewe Record Card. The higher the index, the more valuable the ewe, provided she also has desirable physical characteristics.

Lamb Index

Your Ewe Record Card also provides space for a lamb index. Although this isn't as commonly used as the ewe index, it can be another valuable tool in selecting lambs. Several states are using the following method of computing the lamb index:

Lamb index equals three times the side wool staple length measured in centimeters, plus weight of the lamb adjusted to 120 days. If the lamb was born as a single, 7 points are added; if born as a twin and raised as a twin, 14 points are added.

Health, Veterinary Records

This form makes your Ewe Record Card a self-contained complete record for your flock management program. Record all health information which will prove valuable to you and your veterinarian. This can also serve as a culling and breeding guide.

Success Depends On Your Records

The success of your sheep program will depend to a great extent upon the kind of records you keep. Don't expect amazing results the first year, however. In fact, it may take 5 or 6 years to fully realize significant improvements for keeping good records.

Chapter 48

Disease Management
Of Your Sheep Flock

THIS ANALYSIS of critical sheep diseases can help you determine how best to cope with these particular kinds of problems.

Enteritis

This also relates to scours in lambs.

Stage of Growth: Lambs from birth to 3 weeks. Usually due to damp, wet jugs or yards and E. coli.

Prevention: Clipping udder and crotch of ewes prior to lambing. Make sure that all lambs get colostrum (first milk) right after birth.

Treatment: Place lamb or ewe in dry quarters. Wash udder with a mild chlorine solution. Give lamb an electrolyte solution.

Drug Withholding Time: None.

Overeating Disease

This is also know as clostridium perfringens.

Stage of Growth: This disease affects lambs from birth to market weight.

Prevention: Vaccinate ewes prior to lambing and lambs at 2 and 6 weeks of age.

Treatment: Antitoxin.

Drug Withholding Time: None.

Lamb Pneumonia

Stage of Growth: It hits lambs from 2 weeks to 2 months of age.

Prevention: Treat ewes prior to lambing with 12% sodium sulfamethazine; Mix 1 gal. in 120 gal. of water. Treat for 5 days, then remove for 2 days and then treat again for 2 days.

Treatment: Inject Penicillin or Tetracycline.

Drug Withholding Time: None.

Sore Mouth

Sore mouth is caused by a virus and the disease is called Contagious Ecthyma. It is readily transmitted to humans, so take the necessary precautions.

Stage of Growth: Ewes and lambs are affected by sores on their lips, gums and tongue.

Prevention: Vaccination.

Treatment: Apply tincture of iodine to all sores.

Drug Withholding Time: None.

Mastitis

This is also called Blue Bag in sheep.

Stage of Growth: Shortly after birth to weaning, ewes will have udders that are caked, swollen and sore.

Prevention: This disease is usually due to filth in jugs or paddocks.

Treatment: Treat with mastitis infusions designed for cattle.

Drug Withholding Time: None.

Lambing Paralysis

This is also known as Ketosis.

Stage of Growth: Before or after lambing. It frequently occurs with ewes carrying twins.

Prevention: Feed ewes so they gain 30 lbs. during pregnancy. Don't allow ewes to become fat. Start with grain at the beginning of pregnancy, then gradually increase up to 1 to 1 1/2 lbs. of grain per day.

Treatment: Intravenous injections of sugar solutions.

Drug Withholding Time: None.

White Muscle Disease

Stage of Growth: Lambs 1 to 3 wks. after birth. This is due to a deficiency in selenium.

Prevention: Inject ewes with 5 mg selenium 4 weeks prior to lambing. Provide selenium-fortified salt or a mineral mixture the year round.

Treatment: Inject lambs with 1/4 to 1/2 mg of selenium at 1 or 2 days of age.

Drug Withholding Time: None.

Vibriosis Chlamydia

Stage of Growth: Abortions occur during gestation.

Prevention: Vaccinate with Vibrio-Chlamydia vaccine.

Treatment: At first sign of outbreak, put your entire flock of pregnant ewes on an antibiotic-containing feed. Follow your veterinarian's recommendations.

Drug Withholding Time: None.

Listeriosis

This is also called "Circling Disease."

Stage of Growth: This is usually a more frequent

problem with the older ewes in your flock.

Prevention: The problem usually occurs when ewes are fed silage. In fact, this organism tends to thrive in silage.

Treatment: None is known.

Drug Withholding Time: None.

Foot Rot

This is also called Pododermatitis.

Stage of Growth: It affects all ages of sheep and lambs.

Prevention: Trim all feet. Soak (foot bath) all feet in a zinc sulfate solution. Do not buy sheep from unknown or infected flocks. A vaccine is now available as a preventive, but its effectiveness is not known.

Treatment: Provide footbaths consisting of 8 lbs. zinc sulfate mixed in 10 gal. of water.

Drug Withholding Time: None.

Epididymitis

This is known as Brucellosis in rams.

Stage of Growth: It affects rams from 8 weeks old to maturity.

Prevention: Palpate epididymis and testicle. Determine if this is the problem with a semen culture and serological testing.

Treatment: None.

Drug Withholding Time: None.

Chlamydial, Endemic Abortion

Stage of Growth: Pregnant ewes.

Prevention: Vaccination of ewes before breeding.

Treatment: Tetracycline in case of outbreak.

Drug Withholding Time: 30 days.

Internal Parasites

Stage of Growth: It affects lambs at 4 weeks of age and other sheep regardless of age.

Prevention: For periodic deworming:

1. Drench 1 week prior to lambing.
2. Drench before turning lambs out to pasture.
3. Drench again in 30 days.
4. Drench ewe replacements at the same time.
5. Drench before breeding.

Check with your veterinarian for using an approved dewormer.

Treatment: Use routine deworming on a regularly scheduled basis.

Chapter 49

A Health Program For Your Flock Of Sheep

THIS HEALTH management program is based on following a February lambing program.

January

Health

Vaccinate ewes with Clostridium perfringens C&D 6 and 2 weeks prior to lambing. Inject with selenium. Deworm before lambing.

Nutrition

Offer 4 to 5 mg of salt and mineral per ewe per day and 2 lbs. of grain per ewe per day. Have commercial lamb milk replacer on hand for orphan lambs.

Management

Shear face, udder and crotch of ewes before lambing. See that lambs get colostrum (first milk).

February

Health

Keep ewes and lambs in dry, well-ventilated pens. Don't allow bedding to get wet. For scouring lambs, give a lamb electrolyte solution obtained from your veterinarian.

Nutrition

Provide all the hay that ewes will eat plus 2 lbs. grain per ewe per day. Provide a 15% to 16% protein creep ration for lambs.

Management

Keep ewes and lambs in pens for 1 or 2 days. Warm all chilled lambs. Dock all lambs at 2 or 3 days of age. Castrate at the same time.

March

Health

Shear and treat for ticks. Vaccinate lambs for enterotoxemia (overeating) in the armpit area. Check all feet for foot rot.

Nutrition

Creep feed lambs. Feed 4 to 5 lbs. hay per ewe per day; 1 or 2 lbs. grain per ewe per day.

Management

Identify all ewes to be culled.

April

Health

Wean early lambs. Deworm ewes. If foot rot appears, trim every affected foot. Provide a footbath of 8 lbs. zinc sulfate mixed in 10 gal. of water.

Nutrition

Reduce grain during the sixth or seventh week after lambing.

Management

Take ewes away from lambs—leaving the lambs in familiar paddocks.

May

Health

Check lambs for coccidiosis (scours and loss of weight). Damp, wet pens often lead to coccidiosis problems. Watch for bloat on pasture.

Nutrition

Provide needed minerals and salt. Self-feed lambs.

Management

Select oldest, heaviest twin lambs for replacement purposes.

June

Health

Revaccinate 40 to 50 lb. lambs for enterotoxemia. Deworm ewes and ewe replacements.

Nutrition

Check on pasture quantity and quality.

Management

Check on pastures. Market early lambs if they weigh over 100 lbs.

July

Health

Keep areas cool where you house sheep. Deworm.

Nutrition

Reduce roughage to only 20% in the finishing ration.

Management

Sell the remainder of your lambs.

August

Health

Check ewes for foot rot and maggot infestations.

Nutrition

Rotate pastures. Start ewes on a flushing ration between Aug. 20 and 30.

Management

If possible, expose ewes to rams in lots or fields keeping a fence between them.

September

Health

Vaccinate all ewes for vibriosis. Repeat in 2 weeks.

Nutrition

Cease feeding a flushing ration. Feed rams in daytime.

Management

Turn rams in with ewes only at night. Equip your rams with paint marking harnesses. Use a different color paint every other day.

October

Health

Check ewes daily. Complete the breeding season by Oct. 1.

Nutrition

Change pastures if possible.

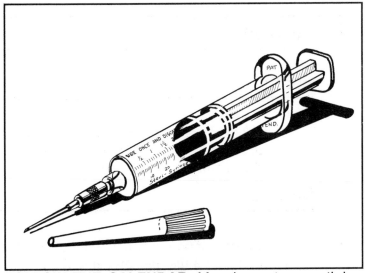

FOLLOW THE CALENDAR. Mapping out a month-by-month health and management program can help you be be sure all work is done on time with your flock of sheep.

November

Health

Pregnancy check your ewes. If abortions occur, rush a fresh fetus to diagnostic laboratory for analysis.

Nutrition

Feed supplemental hay if pastures are short.

Management

Keep a "teaser" animal with your ewes. Cull all ewes that are still in heat.

December

Health

Check ewes for lice and ticks. Shear if adequate housing is available, then treat with Co-Ral or Malathion.

Nutrition

If hay is of poor quality, feed grain. Starting slowly, feed 1 or 2 lbs. per ewe per day.

Management

Prepare lambing jugs. Dry bedding and well-ventilated quarters are a "must."

Chapter 50

Making Injections In Your Sheep

BEFORE MAKING any kind of injection or administering any drugs to your sheep, be sure to read the medication label carefully. Before going ahead, read and be sure you understand the cautions, proper dosage, frequency of administration and recommended method of administration.

In this chapter, we will give you detailed information on how to make the type of injections recommended for sheep.

Intramuscular Injections

An intramuscular injection is made through the skin and subcutaneous tissue, directly into the muscle of the animal. Absorption is very rapid in this case. It is commonly used in sheep, cattle and swine.

Equipment Needed

- A 25 or 50-cc veterinary syringe.

- Hypodermic needle, 16 gauge, 3/4 in. long.

- Scissors or clippers.

- 70% rubbing alcohol compound or other equally

effective antiseptic for disinfecting the skin and bottle stopper.

• The medication to be given.

Preparing Your Equipment

Clean and disinfect the needles and syringe by boiling in water for 20 minutes.

Areas Of Injection

An intramuscular injection is made directly into the animal's muscle tissue or meat. Heavily muscled portions of the body such as the neck, shoulder and hindquarter should be utilized. In small animals, such as sheep, not more than 10 to 15 cc of medicine should be injected in any one spot. Where the dosage to be given is large, this can be done by distributing the dosage in 15-cc amounts into the heavy muscles of the neck, shoulder or hindquarter on both sides of the animal.

Preparing The Animals

Restrain the animal by the best means available. Clip the wool from the area where the injection is to be given. Swab the clipped areas vigorously with alcohol or an other equally effective antiseptic.

Inserting Needle, Making Injection

Fill the syringe with the medication to be given, using a separate needle for filling. Disinfect the rubber stopper before inserting the needle into the bottle.

Insert a previously disinfected needle deeply into

the muscle tissue with a quick thrust. Observe the hub of the needle for a moment. If blood begins to flow out of the needle, it is probably in a blood vessel and the needle should be withdrawn and reinserted in a different direction. Attach the syringe to the needle, then inject the medication slowly.

After the medication has been injected, remove the

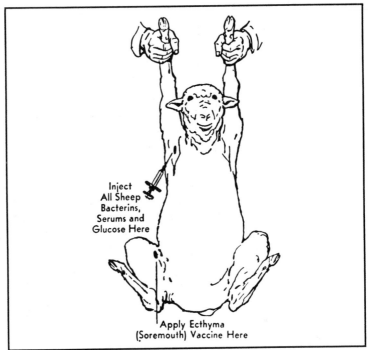

SHEEP INJECTIONS. Intramuscular injections are made directly into the muscle tissue or meat portions of the body such as the neck and shoulder.

A subcutaneous injection is made beneath the skin and the muscle tissue. The recommended areas of injection are in those places where the skin is loose, particularly on the sides of the neck and behind the shoulder. In this illustration, the axillary space is being used for this type of injection. This is the space between the foreleg and the chest wall which will correspond to the armpit in man. Bacterins, serums and glucose solutions are injected here.

needle still attached to the syringe and massage the area with cotton soaked in alcohol to spread the medication through the muscle tissue. This procedure should be repeated in each injection area until the full recommended dose has been given.

Subcutaneous Injections

A subcutaneous injection is made into the layers of tissue beneath the skin. As with the intramuscular injection, this method is also commonly used in sheep, cattle and swine.

First, read the directions for making an intramuscular injection. The equipment needed, its preparation and preparation of the animal are the same as for the intramuscular injection.

A subcutaneous injection is an injection made beneath the skin and the muscle tissue. The recommended areas for injection are places where the skin is loose, particularly on the sides of the neck and behind the shoulder. In sheep, the axillary space is frequently used for subcutaneous injection. The axillary space lies between the foreleg and the chest wall, corresponding to a man's armpit.

To make the injection, pinch a fold of skin between the thumb and fingers (This is not necessary if the axillary space is used). Insert the needle under the fold in a direction approximately parallel to the surface of the body. When the needle is inserted in this manner, medication will be delivered underneath the skin and the muscles. Observe the same precautions regarding clipping and disinfecting the skin as outlined in the section dealing with intramuscular injections.

Chapter 51

Properly Managing Your Dairy Goats

DUE TO THE increased interest in goats throughout the United States and the lack of essential information on production of goats, the following facts on goat production have been assembled for the goat raiser or person thinking of getting started.

The goat, Capra hircus, has been domesticated for thousands of years and is regarded in many countries of the world as the poor man's cow. It is becoming increasingly popular in the United States as a source of meat and milk. As a result, there has been a sharp increase in the price of goats.

Anatomy Of The Goat

Goats are herbivores and have the typical four-sectioned stomach of a ruminant. Goats with horns are socially dominant over those that do not have them, but the polled characteristic is genetically dominant.

Although the presence of wattles is also due to a dominant gene, they serve no useful purpose and many people clip them at birth. In the young kid, they are soft. In mature animals, the hairs are stiffer and are arranged in a spiral pattern around the wattle so it resembles a bottle brush. Wattles are usually placed symmetrically on the neck, but occasionally may be found at the angle of the jaw or up close to the ears. Beards occur in some individuals of both sexes and develop during the first year or so of life.

Goats are cloven hoofed. There is no gland between the digits and no infraorbital or inguinal glands.

Although the goat appears to have a split upper lip, there is actually only a line and not a split in the skin. They are aged by the appearance of the eight incisor teeth on the lower jaw (there are none on the top jaw). Kids have eight small milk incisors.

At around 1 year of age, the two permanent central incisors erupt. At 1 1/2 to 2 years, four permanent teeth are present. At 2 1/2 to 3 years, six teeth are present. At 3 1/2 to 4 years, all eight teeth are visible and fully grown—the animal is said to have a 'full mouth'. Very old goats lose teeth and are called "broken mouthed".

Goats are usually fairly thin, the ribs and backbone are easily felt and a hollow exists in the upper flank. Fat goats are rare. A large abdomen in a non-pregnant animal indicates she has a good capacity for food and that hopefully she will be able to eat more and therefore give more milk.

Goats that are well cared for and fed properly have a life span of 8 to 12 years, sometimes living up to 20 years. They have a normal temperature of 102 to 104 degrees F. Castration should be done when kids are 1 to 4 weeks of age.

Anatomical defects with goats include:

• Long weak pasterns on the legs.

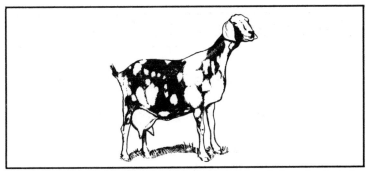

GOOD MANAGEMENT IS CRITICAL. A herd of dairy goats can be very profitable, providing essential health and management practices are carried out at the correct times.

- Undershot jaw (the lower jaw is too long for the teeth to touch the pad).

- Supernumeray teats.

- Double teats.

- Teats that are too big.

- Teats that are too small.

Other problems include myotonia, a non-lethal hereditary defect of the muscle fibers. It causes the goat's legs to stiffen and the animal to often fall in response to sudden noise or movement. Affected animals are known as "fainting" or "nervous" goats.

Goat udders have very large milk cisterns and teat canals which can store a lot of milk. However, they can also collapse dramatically when emptied.

Musk glands on the head are most developed in the mature buck. It is from these glands that a large proportion of the powerful buck smell comes. Females are called does and the young are called kids. Doelings and bucklings are immature animals.

Physiology Of The Goat

Normal Lifespan: 8-12 years.

Body Temperature: 102 to 104 degrees F.

Blood Volume: 7% of body weight.

Packed Cell Volume: 30% to 35%.

Urine Characteristics: A pH 7-8 is normal, but it will be lower during lactation.

Fecal Characteristics: Firm dark pellets, 1/2 to 1 centimeter in diameter. On lush pasture, they become softer and less formed.

Milk Composition: 87% water, 3% to 5% butterfat and 3% protein.

Passive Immunity: None to the fetus. Transfer occurs via the colostrum for 1 or 2 days.

Goat's Milk

An ordinary doe will probably give 3 to 4 pts. of milk per day during her lactation. High producing animals give over 4 qts. a day and up to 3,000 lbs. per. year. The record 305 day lactation for a Toggenberg goat is 5,750 lbs. of milk. Although the butterfat content is the same or greater than cows' milk, the fat globules are smaller and therefore the cream does not separate as easily. The curds are also smaller, softer and easier to digest than those in cows' milk. This probably contributes to the legendary ability of goat's milk to cure many diseases, particularly those of the gastro-intestinal tract.

The milk sometimes develops a peculiar taste which can be attributed to various causes:

- Strong flavored food in the diet.

- Indigestion and temporary acidosis.

- The use of plastic milking pails.

- Cooling the milk too slowly, especially in an odoriferous area.

- Covering the milk can while cooling it.

- Overdeveloped musk glands on the head of the female.

- Housing females too close to bucks.

Goats are creatures of habit and are generally fed grain at milking time to induce milk let down. A great deal of affection seems to develop for which-ever creature delivers the milk—a kid, human or even a foster animal.

The occasional goat that kicks while being milked can be controlled by tying a soft cotton rope tightly around the abdomen just in front of the udder.

Goats can be very noisy, especially the Nubian breed. If animals are housed alone, they become lonely and complain loudly. This can be a serious problem in a confined area. If young kids make a lot of noise, they are said to be "blatting."

Breeds Of Goats

Saanen

This is a white dairy goat weighing up to 200 lbs. which generally enjoys a quiet temperament. Beards and wattles are common in both sexes. The yellow stains often seen on these animals are caused by the buck urinating on himself.

Toggenberg

This is a brown dairy goat, varying in color from milk chocolate to dark chocolate. They always have pale legs and facial stripes. Beards and wattles are often present. Normal weight is around 150 lbs. The face has a tendency to be dished.

French Alpine

This very alert looking dairy goat has striking color patterns. Black and white or sandy and grey are common colors. The ears are erect and wattles and beards are sometimes present. Two other Alpine breeds exist in the United States in small numbers, the Swiss and the Rock.

Nubian

This breed differs from the previous three since it hails not from Europe, but from the Middle East and Africa. It is the only breed having long bell-shaped drooping ears and a Roman nose. Wattles and beards are often seen. This goat is frequently spotted and multi-colored. These animals tend to be slab-sided with less "gut" than other breeds.

Milk production is slightly lower for Nubians than other dairy breeds, but butterfat content is higher.

This is probably the most vocal goat of all. This buck has white legs, but he has usually urinated on them and they are thus stained yellow brown.

La Mancha

This breed has short or nonexistent ear pinnae. These dairy goats are becoming quite popular.

Angora

This is not a dairy animal and is kept solely for its fleece, known as mohair. The animals are usually clipped in the spring before they normally shed their coats and again in the fall. Fleece weight from quality bucks is around 10 to 15 lbs. The length of the outer fibers is around 10 in. The underhair is known as kemp and is not desirable because it will not take dyes as well as the mohair.

These goats are usually found in the dry regions of the Southwest and do not thrive as well in areas of high rainfall. They are quite small and usually only have one kid each year. The ears may be either erect or drooping.

Mexican Goats

These are commonly mixed crossbreds which are found through the Southwestern area of the United States. They are typically similar to mohair-producing goats.

Pygmy West African Dwarf Goats

These very small goats weigh only 40 to 50 lbs. at maturity. Since their milking ability is not high, they are generally kept as pets or used as research animals.

Grade Goats

These have only one parent who is a registered pedigree animal.

Scrub Goats

These are the lowest level of goat society. They may represent any number of grade and/or crossbreeding programs.

Registering Purebred Goats

The American Goat Society acts as a registry for purebred goats. The American Dairy Goat Assn. registers both grades and purebreds. After three generations of using purebred males on grade females, it is possible to introduce enough purebred blood in a head to make the resulting grades eligible for entry in the purebred register of the American Dairy Goat Assn. However, they remain identified forever as ex-grades by being called, for example, American Saanen instead of Saanen only.

Handling Goats

Although they are gregarious and like the company of each other and humans, goats will not stay in flocks and follow each other like sheep. This makes it much more difficult to drive a group of goats. Single animals are best handled with a leather collar, as they can be trained to walk on a leash.

Horned goats are dangerous to each other and people. Unless they are extremely trustworthy, they should be restrained by the horns, although they do not like it. This gives them no opportunity to swing their heads and use the horns as hooks.

When alarmed, goats snort, stamp their fore feet, flatten their tails up over their backs and raise the hair along the spine. The presence of dogs often makes them very agitated and difficult to handle.

On the whole, goats are friendly, individualistic

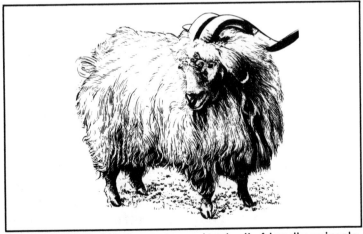

BE CAREFUL. While goats are basically friendly animals, horned goats can be very dangerous. They can injure you and also damage equipment and buildings with their horns.

animals that respond to affection and petting. Threats and brute force have little effect and often provoke defiance. There are a few mean goats that will charge and hit you on the back of the knees. Never turn your back on this kind.

Identifying Goats

For identification purposes, tattooing the ears is the most permanent method. The American Goat Society requires that the right ear be tattooed with the owner's assigned letters and the left ear be tattooed with a code letter corresponding to the year of birth. The breed organization does not specify the tattooing procedure.

Ear tags can be used, but once in a while they will work loose and fall out. It is not safe to rely on the color of kids for identification since some change coat patterns and color intensity as they mature.

Managing Your Goat Herd

A number of key management practices should be followed to have a successful goat operation.

Housing

Animals can be housed in groups with 15 sq. ft. per goat. If housed in individual boxes or stanchions, they should be within sight or sound of other goats since one goat kept alone gets very lonely and very noisy. They hate getting wet and will not thrive if they have to sleep on damp bedding. Housing does not have to be heated, but it should be draft proof.

Fences should be at least 4 ft. high (5 ft. for males) and made of wood or heavy gauge woven wire. Goats stand on their hind legs and break down or scramble over lesser types of fences. They love to climb on top of things. Trees in your pasture must be protected by wrapping wire netting around the trunk; otherwise the bark will be peeled off. Two or three strands of electric fence will control goats.

Dehorning

If the hair curls in a rosette over the hornbud area and the skin is not freely movable, horns are going to grow. There are two cornual nerves supplying each horn on the lateral side, so any local anesthesia should be infiltrated below the lateral horn base. The goats will complain as much with the local anesthetic as if dehorning had been done without it!

The electrically heated dehorning iron is the best instrument to use. A modification involving a solid copper rod screwed into the heating iron and hollowed out to form a cutting edge works very well. If you can pop the horn bud off, then the horn tissue has been adequately destroyed. To be absolutely sure, the iron may be rotated around the outer rim of skin. During dehorning, the musk glands on the buck, caudal and medial to the horn, can be destroyed by touching them with the iron.

Young kids can also be dehorned by rubbing a caustic paste on the bud after the hair has been clipped off. However, this can be dangerous since the kid may get caustic solution running into its eyes or it may rub its head on the dam's udder while nursing.

Painting the horn buds with a collodion solution is no longer a popular method of dehorning.

Any chicken-heartedness on the part of the operator with the hot iron will cause the regrowth of unsightly scars and deformed horns which may curve back into the head.

Dehorning adult goats is a bloody mess. There is some risk involved since the frontal sinus is small and the horn is quite close to the brain. If the horn is held or twisted, the skull may fracture. Horns should be cut 1/4 in. below the horn/skin junction.

Obstetrical wire, meat saws and scoop type dehorners have all been used to dehorn goats. The sinus cavity is usually opened in mature animals and this operation should not be done during fly season because of the danger of maggots in the wound. "Elastrator" bands, used for castrating animals, have also been used for dehorning. They should be applied as far down the horn as possible. It takes 6 to 8 weeks for the horn to drop off due to reduced blood supply and there will be some discomfort.

Trimming The Feet

Goat's feet grow very fast and need trimming periodically. This can be done in a standing position, picking up one foot at a time. If a foot won't cooperate, lay the goat on its side, with the operator behind the goat's back and with one knee on its neck. Goats wriggle a lot if sat on their rump like sheep. A useful, cheap trimming instrument is a pair of garden clippers, but the correct instrument to use is a set of hoof shears.

Buck Management

Mature bucks smell so bad that they should be kept as far away as possible and downwind from both lactating does and humans. The odor is worse during the breeding season, although the intensity of individual bucks varies from year to year. Nubian bucks are reputed to be the least smelly.

Each musk gland on top of the head is about 2 centimeters square. The overlying skin is hypertrophied and wrinkled. Destroying the glands during dehorning reduces but does not eliminate the odor.

The buck will also urinate down the back of the forelegs and over the neck and beard, making the skin bald and thickened. Shearing off all long hair, scrubbing the head daily with 70% alcohol or hexachlorophene solution and washing off the urine may reduce the smell a little. However, nothing will eliminate it, except castration. Nothing will get it off equipment or buildings and it takes a long time to wear off your skin if you make the mistake of touching the animal.

During the breeding season, bucks often refuse to eat if there are does nearby. If fact, they may fret, worry and eat so little that their growth will be permanently stunted. Bucks may be sexually mature at 2 or 3 months of age, especially if born in the summer. Doe kids should thus be raised separately from buck kids.

The easiest time to castrate a male is when it is small with the Burdizzo bloodless emasculatome. When using this method, it is important not to let the cord slip sideways. Using a Burdizzo with side clamps will avoid this problem. Castrated bucks are called wethers and grow larger than a buck.

Feeding, Watering

While it is generally said that 6 or 8 goats will eat as much as one cow, a goat can have a phenomenal appetite. Some have been reported as eating up to 10% of their body weight in dry matter daily. By comparison, the average cow eats only 4% of its body weight in dry matter daily. The goat's capacity for eating is partly due to the fact that its rumen is extremely large in relation to its body size.

To keep a goat for a year, you will need at least 10 to 14 bales of hay (500 to 700 lb.) and good summer pasture. In addition, grain should be fed at approximately 1/2 lb. per pound of milk produced in winter and 1/4 lb. per pound of milk produced in summer when the animal is on pasture. Goats that do not go out to grass should get as much hay as they want and enough grain to keep them in good condition, generally 1/2 to 1 lb. per day.

Great care should be taken not to suddenly increase the amount of grain fed as this can make the goat severely ill.

As a rule, goats don't like dusty, fine ground food and prefer coarse chunks or whole grains. They are messy hay feeders. Once they have dropped hay on the floor, only starvation will make them pick it up again.

They prefer brush, flowers and weeds to grass. As a result, they will eventually destroy any shrubs or small trees growing in your pastures.

In winter, goats will drink more water if it is warmed slightly. In the summer, they prefer fresh water which is offered frequently. They should also have loose trace mineral salt available.

Breeding Goats

Goats generally come into heat first during the fall of the same year in which they are born. Some may be precocious and conceive as early as 3 months; pygmy goats, for example, may do this. Doelings are usually bred when they reach 65 to 80 lbs. Some people feel breeding a goat in the first year will stunt it while others say if the goat is well grown and fed properly then it does not make a difference.

The breeding season usually runs from September to February, although pygmies may start earlier and finish later. Some does, particularly Nubians, will breed at any time, although not every buck is willing to breed outside of the normal breeding season.

They are polyoestrous, coming into heat approximately every 20 to 21 days while pygmies may have a 24-day cycle. Heat lasts about 2 days and can be recognized by the following signs:

- The doe is very persistent and noisy.

- She urinates a lot.

- She swishes her tail.

- There may be a dropoff in milk production.

- She rides and is ridden by other goats.

- She is found staying close to the buck pen.

They are usually bred towards the end of the heat period, close to ovulation. If the goats are milking, they are not allowed to run with the buck because they will pick up the smell in their milk.

The Kids Are Coming

Gestation averages 150 days with a range of 144 to 157 days. Pseudopregnancy occasionally occurs and the goat eventually delivers a large volume of fluid. She does not appear to suffer any ill effects and the succeeding pregnancy is usually normal.

Twin kids are more common than singles while triplets are not rare. Birth weight varies from 5 to 9 lbs. according to how many there are in the uterus. There is no problem with hermaphroditism due to placental sharing between male and female kids. However, genetic hermaphroditism does exist in homozygous polled females due to probable linkage of the poll and intersex genes.

Signs of impending parturition are relaxation of the pelvic ligaments, a raising of the tail head, sagging of the abdomen with an increase in the size of the flank hollow, tightening of the udder and swelling of the vulva.

Goats usually give birth lying down, but occasionally deliver standing up—watch that the kid is not dropped into the water bucket because it could drown.

The placenta is passed within 4 hours and cases of retained placentae are very unusual. If it is necessary to assist a doe during a difficult birth, the goat will resort to agonized bleating. They do not take pain well.

Most people take kids away from the mother immediately and feed them colostrum from a bottle. This causes less emotional trauma than doing it a few days later. If the kids are not taken from the mother when she goes out to graze, she will leave

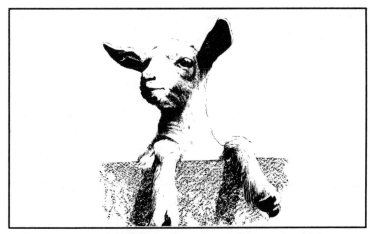

WEAN THEM EARLY. Many producers take kids away from their mothers immediately after birth and feed them colostrum milk right from a bottle. This helps gets kids off to a fast start in life and also reduces the trauma and concerns of taking them away from mother at a later date.

the kids in a secluded spot and they remain quite content. A few does will come into heat immediately after parturition and may conceive.

Young kids are traditionally reared on goat's milk for an extended period of 4 to 6 months. They could be fed on milk replacer or whole cows' milk, but should always receive goat colostrum for 3 days. They usually do better if fed goat's milk for a week.

They will drink 1 1/2 to 2 pts. of milk each day in divided feedings. Wean them when they are eating grain properly.

A goat should be milked for 305 days and then rest for 6 to 8 weeks before delivering. However, a common fault is a short lactation period and some don't even last 6 months. By selection, it is even possible to get goats to milk for 2 years and only breed them biennially.

Drug Administration

Worming preparations and other medications are often given by mouth in the form of liquid, known as a "drench." A small plastic syringe can be used, but a bigger one such as 30 cc is difficult to use because the goat chews on it too much.

A metal dosing syringe is convenient, but a commercial drenching gun is even easier to use. The goat should be backed into a corner and its head held in a normal position. The drenching instrument should be pushed into the gap between the molars and the incisors, then directed back towards the throat. If the animal's head is pulled too high, it may not swallow properly and the fluid will go down the trachea and cause inhalation pneumonia. Goats are harder to dose than sheep because the neck is longer and they wriggle more.

Some drugs come in the form of boluses and have to be given with a balling gun. Push the balling gun into the gap in the side of the mouth and to the back of the mouth. If it is only pushed halfway back, the goat will invariably spit out the bolus. Don't put your fingers in a goat's mouth; their molars are extremely sharp and jagged.

Internal Parasites

Several critical parasite problems are commonly found in herds of goats.

Moniezia

This is the common cestode or tapeworm. The segments can easily be seen in the feces and are often mistaken for maggots. While these worms are not regarded as being very significant, it may be necessary to remove them from the goat for aesthetic reasons.

Check with your veterinarian for the wormer of choice in treating tapeworm infestations.

Coccidial Oocysts

These parasites can be found in practically all goats, but the clinical signs of disease usually are only seen in young animals. Kids kept in conditions where there is a lot of fecal contamination of food and water may develop heavy infections. This may cause a severe hemmorrhagic enteris which is often fatal if left untreated.

Coccidiostats should be placed in kid rations as soon as they start eating. Continue feeding until the kids reach 4 months of age.

Lungworms

These are common in goats. Muellerins spp. live in the lung parenchyma and do not cause much damage or any clinical signs.

Dictyocaulus is much less common, fortunately. Since it is a very dangerous parasite, living in the bronchioles and interfering with respiration, it can have fatal consequences. Tramisol is very effective as a lungworm treatment.

External Parasites

Goats are hosts to a variety of lice, both blood suckers and skin chewers. These problems appear more numerous in winter in confined animals and can contribute to a loss in condition. Spraying with an insecticide is more effective than using powder. In either case, treatment should be repeated in 10 to 14 days.

Undernutrition Concerns

There is a common misconception that goats can live on cigarette ends, tin cans and newspapers. While they do have strange tastes, they are also very particular about what they eat. They don't like dirty, dusty or moldy feed. Hay that has fallen on the floor will never be eaten. It is possible for a goat to become half starved, with food in front of it, just because it doesn't like what is being offered.

Overeating Problems

This problem is as dangerous to the goat as to any other ruminant animal. It is a mistake to think that because they like grain they can eat as much as they want. If it is necessary that a goat should eat a lot, the amount should be increased gradually every day.

Mild overeating causes indigestion and diarrhea; heavy overeating causes grain-poisoning, acidosis and often death. A further complication is entero-toxemia due to Clostridium perfringens. It is almost always fatal and there is no treatment.

Chapter 52

A Health Program
For Your Dairy Goats

GOATS ARE BECOMING increasingly popular
and more and more herds are developing throughout the country. In many cases, developers of these
herds have not owned or managed animals before.
Consequently, they are not always conscious of
their responsibilities in owning animals, particularly animals whose products are used for human
consumption.

In only 7 years, the number of owners of purebred
dairy goats in this country increased from 900 to
3,900 owners. The average herd is composed of only
12 goats; yet some herds number up to 700 to 800
head.

World wide, more people drink goat's milk than
cow's milk. The price of fairly good quality milk
goats runs $100 to $200 each. However, purebred
mothers can sell for as much as $1,000 a head.

Critical Disease Concerns

The major diseases of goats can be discussed as one
would analyze small ruminant animals such as
sheep. A discussion of goats and their management
follows the same pattern.

Brucellosis And Tuberculosis

Dairy goat herds are seldom infected with either disease. Yet animals should be tested for both diseases before being added to your herd. Since both diseases are transmitted to humans, your animals should be found free of these diseases by testing if milk is to be sold for human consumption.

Caseous Lymphadinitis

One of the most serious diseases of goats, it also can be transmitted to man. It is caused by an organism called Corynebacterium pseudotuberculosis that affects lymph glands, producing abscesses. For every lymph gland found to be infected, ten other glands are hidden. This disease is the main reason why goats become thin and die.

Kids must be separated from adults at birth and fed colostrum milk from clean udders. Adding 100 grams per ton of oxytetracycline or chlortetracycline to all grain fed to young animals is also helpful in controlling this problem. Some herd owners are even using a special bacterin made from infections within the herd.

Enterotoxemia

This disease is most frequently found in well managed herds. Goats of all ages are susceptible to clostridium perfringens type B, C and D. Sudden death in young kids and even in older animals can occur when there is a change in grain rations, hay or pasture. All animals over 1 month of age should be given polyvalent Cl. perfringens toxoid in two doses at least 2 weeks apart. This should be repeated annually.

Mastitis

If goat's milk is to be used for human consumption, the same rules for quality milk production used in dairy herds should apply to goat herds. Sanitizing the udder prior to milking, washing your hands between milkers and teat dipping after milking are strongly recommended.

Goat owners are also urged to have their veterinarian culture the milk from infected glands and determine antibiotic sensitivity. Determining the drug of choice in this way is mandatory for successful treatment. It must also be remembered that every drug is not going to prove successful as a treatment. Milk from infected glands should also be discarded for at least 96 hours following treatment.

Internal Parasites

Like sheep, goats are almost always parasitized. Check with your veterinarian for the drug of choice which will rid animals of lungworms and other internal parasites. However, the dosage should be watched very carefully. Goats should be wormed at least twice a year—more often if pastures are short and overstacked or paddocks are contaminated.

Pneumonia

One of the biggest problems with goat management is that owners tend to house their animals in "tight" buildings. If condensation occurs on building walls, then pneumonia almost always develops. Goats will actually remain healthier if allowed to run in free housing and are not confined within a tight building.

Dehorning Goats

Male goats smell while females do not. However, females actually like the male goat's odors. Much of this odor comes from the musk glands found around the base of the horn. Billygoats usually smell because they urinate all over themselves. Coupled with the odor from the musk glands, this is sometimes difficult for some people to tolerate.

Goats under 2 weeks of age can be easily dehorned. The area for dehorning should be blocked with 1 to 2 cc of a local anesthetic and a hot (cherry red) soldering iron. Clip around the base of the horns so you can see the musk glands, then apply the hot iron to both the horn bud and the musk glands.

Foot Rot

The same procedure for handling foot rot in sheep can also be used with goats. All hooves must be examined and those with excess growth will need trimming. Goats having hooves with dry rot or abscesses should be allowed to stand in a foot bath of copper sulfur for 20 minutes. Repeat for 2 weeks.

Goats Versus Cattle

Disease spread in goats follows the same principles that exist with cattle. Infected animals are a threat to other animals. Diseases can be spread by semen from an infected male. Brucellosis, tuberculosis, Johne's Disease and viral diseases can be transmitted from the infected male to susceptible females.

Chapter 53

Horse Diseases And Management Practices

HERE ARE some of the most common disease problems which can affect your horses.

Tetanus

The vaccination of horses against tetanus is highly recommended. Tetanus antitoxin is given to injured animals which are not immunized with tetanus toxoid. Toxoid may also be given to injured animals, since there is a possible risk in routinely using a tetanus antitoxin.

The initial immunization consists of the first injection followed by a second injection 2 to 4 weeks later. An annual booster should also be administered. Foals are first vaccinated at 2 or 3 months.

Eastern, Western Equine Encephalomyelitis

Vaccination is recommended by veterinarians in most states. An initial vaccination is usually given in the spring (April or May) followed by a second injection 7 to 14 days later. Both injections should be repeated annually. Foals are first immunized at 2 or 3 months of age.

Equine Influenza

Viruses other than flu virus can cause symptoms of influenza. Even after vaccination, an animal can still develop an influenza-like disease. Vaccination against influenza produces variable results.

The initial injection should be followed by a second in 4 to 12 weeks. An annual booster is also recommended. Foals are first vaccinated at 2 or 3 months of age.

Venezuelan Equine Encephalomyelitis

Regulatory authorities place a high priority on vaccination against this disease. Human exposure may also result in an influenza-type infection. Since the disease is not endemic in some states, vaccination is not compulsory.

One injection is given. Research shows the vaccine will not cause pregnant mares to abort.

Duration of immunity is at least 18 months and possibly longer. Foals are vaccinated at 3 months of age. Some states also require horses to be vaccinated for VEE before entry.

Equine Infectious Anemia

No vaccine is available for this disease. An excellent, accurate diagnostic test (Coggin's Test) is routinely performed by certain approved laboratories.

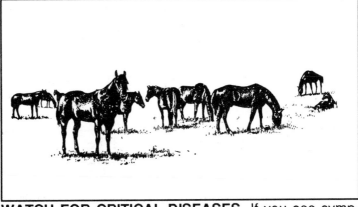

WATCH FOR CRITICAL DISEASES. If you see symptoms developing for any of these diseases in your horses, be sure to consult immediately with your own veterinarian.

All horses exported to Canada require proof of a negative Coggin's test within the previous 6 months. Over 40 states now require horses to be negative to Coggin's test before entry.

Rabies

Vaccination is recommended only in geographic areas where rabies is considered endemic or epizootic. It is a prophylactic vaccination.

An initial injection is followed by a second injection 30 days later. Foals are first vaccinated at 3 months of age. An annual vaccination is recommended.

Strangles (Distemper)

Vaccination against strangles is not recommended under many conditions since some complications may result.

When vaccination is used, the first injection is followed by a second injection 1 week later. A third injection is given 7 days after the second injection.

A yearly re-vaccination is then recommended. Foals are first vaccinated at 3 months of age.

Viral Rhinopneumonitis

This is a viral disease that produces respiratory symptoms in young horses. In older horses, very mild clinical symptoms are experienced with this disease.

Mares which are exposed to this disease during mid-pregnancy will frequently abort during late pregnancy.

An annual vaccination of pregnant mares and show horses is recommended. This intramuscular vaccine should be given after 60 days of pregnancy and again between the fifth and seventh months of pregnancy.

Young show horses and race horses should receive two annual injections 4 to 8 weeks apart. Foals can be vaccinated at 2 or 3 months of age.

Leptospirosis

Vaccination for this disease is recommended only in areas where the disease is endemic.

One injection is given every 6 months. One or two injections are recommended annually and foals are first vaccinated when 3 months old.

Chapter 54

Controlling Internal Parasites In Horses

THERE ARE five classes of internal parasites which most commonly affect horses:

- Large strongyles.

- Small strongyles.

- Ascarids.

- Pinworms.

- Bots.

The large strongyles found in horses are also known as bloodworms, palisade worms or red worms. There are three closely related species that make up this group: Strongyles vulgaris, S. edentatus and S. equinus.

These large strongyles may vary in length from 1/2 to 1 1/2 in. The adult worms attach themselves to the lining of the caecum and colon. The females produce eggs that are passed in the droppings.

Under favorable conditions, larvae develop into an infective stage within 7 days after the eggs are first passed. The larvae are resistant to drying and to low temperatures.

Infection occurs when the larvae contaminate food

or water. Larvae from these three species migrate extensively after entering the intestine before they develop into maturity within the large intestine. Larvae of S. vulgaris commonly migrate to the branches or the mesenteric (intestinal) arteries where they may cause damage and irritation and may result in parasitic aneurism.

Signs Of Infection

Those signs sometimes associated with internal parasitic infections are rough hair coat, weakness, emaciation, colic, chronic cough, stunted growth, diarrhea (sometimes bloody) and tail rubbing.

Unfortunately, an infestation of external parasites may cause some of the same symptoms which are associated with internal parasites. For example, dense populations of lice or ticks on a horse may result in weakness and emaciation; both the tail louse and a pinworm infection can cause tail rubbing. Loss of hair may be due to lice or, in some instances, insect bites.

The success of an internal parasite control program in horses depends upon the choice of the most effective drug and its proper application to the parasite problem. A sustained schedule of treatment is required to reduce the potential of worm populations to subclinical levels. Treatment must be continued if the potential parasitic population is to be held to a low level.

General points of importance which must be kept in mind include:

☛ No single preparation should be used exclusively.

☛ The entire horse population on the premises should be included in any control program.

☛ New additions (permanent or temporary) should be quarantined and treated before being introduced into the resident group of animals. Periodic fecal examinations should be made.

Sanitation Is Critical

Good sanitation should be emphasized. Precautions include routine removal of feces, composting before spreading on pastures, rotation of pastures where possible, keeping feed off the ground, preventing fecal contamination of water, pasturing yearlings and weanlings separately from older horses and properly screening and treating all additions to the herd.

The most serious damage from parasites occurs in young horses during their first 2 years of life. The greatest injury to foals and weanlings is insidious and parasitism results in varying degrees of impaired growth, development and resistance to diseases.

However, some parasites in or on mature horses can cause unthriftiness, weakness and increased susceptibility to disease—even leading to death. Injury to all horses is related primarily to the type and number of parasites present and the length of time over which infection or infestations are acquired.

Recommended Worming—Foals

These practices can help you carry out a successful program for controlling internal parasites.

60 days

Schedule of Administration: 60 days.

Parasites Controlled: Strongyles and ascarids.

120 days

Schedule of Administration: Every 60 days.

Parasites Controlled: Strongyles and ascarids.

180 days

Schedule of Administration: Every 60 days.

Parasites Controlled: Strongyles and ascarids.

220 days

Schedule of Administration: 40 days (Weaned).

Parasites Controlled: Strongyles, ascarids and bots.

December

Schedule of Administration: Weanlings.

Parasites Controlled: Strongyles, ascarids, bots.

February, March

Schedule of Administration: Yearlings.

Parasites Controlled: Strongyles, ascarids and bots.

November, December

Parasites Controlled: Strongyles, ascarids and bots.

Recommended Worming—Mares

You can follow a similar worming program for mares that are either brood and/or barren.

Pregnant

Schedule of Administration: December, January or February.

Parasites Controlled: Strongyles and bots.

Lactating

Schedule of Administration: Aug. 1.

Parasites Controlled: Strongyles and bots.

Post Weaning

Schedule of Administration: Oct. 15.

Parasites Controlled: Strongyles and bots.

Recommended Worming—Stallions

Schedule Of Administration: Based on fecal examination, every 60 days. A count of 50 eggs per gram or more indicates a need for reworming.

Parasites Controlled: Strongyles and bots.

Worm Treatment Recommendations

There are several dewormers on the market which are available in different forms. Some can be placed in the feed while others are available in paste form.

There is some indication that the continuous use of any one horse dewormer can develop resistance against the active ingredient found in a particular product. As a result, the rotation of dewormers is frequently recommended.

Veterinarians frequently use a tube passed through the nostril that reaches into the horse's stomach as a means of effectively administering dewormers.

In view of the effectiveness of some dewormers for certain types of internal parasites and the fact that worm resistance may develop from continuous use of any dewormer, it is recommended that a veterinarian's advice be followed as to the type of dewormer to use and the method of administration.

You will find there are several excellent dewormers on the market which are readily available.

Chapter 55

A Herd Health Program For Horses

HERE IS a month-by-month health management program that you can follow that will result in much better health for your horses.

January, February, March

Deworm all horses, especially pregnant mares at 8 week intervals.

Take care of any dentistry problems according to need.

Test all race, show, sale and breeding horses for equine infectious anemia.

For immunizations, administer Tetanus Toxoid to all horses, especially pregnant mares. Immunize against respiratory diseases such as influenza and Rhinopneumonitis.

For stallions, carry out a semen evaluation. Provide 16 hours of light out of every 24 hours.

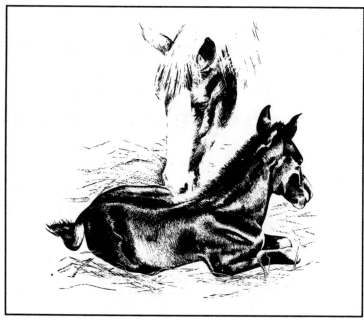

BASIC MANAGEMENT IDEAS PAY OFF. By following this month-by-month health management program as closely as you can, your own horses will be in better shape.

April, May, June

Deworm as needed.

Administer respiratory vaccines as indicated.

Evaluate foals for epiphysitis or limb deviation.

Conduct pregnancy exams at 18 to 23 days, again at 35 days and once more at 50-70 days.

Monitor semen gathering from breeding stallions each week.

Administer Eastern and Western Equine Encephalomyelitis vaccine.

Give PHF vaccine if the need is indicated.

Foals over 2 months of age should receive a Tetanus Toxoid, Eastern and Western Equine Encephalomyelitis vaccine and be dewormed.

July, August, September

Deworm.

Administer immunization boosters as needed.

Evaluate foals for limb and joint soundness.

Reconfirm all pregnancies.

Promote stressless weaning. All foals over 4 months of age should be dewormed and immunizations given as needed. Remove the mares and leave the foals in familiar surroundings.

Adjust nutrition for foals. Feed a 16% protein ration and offer hay and pasture free choice. Provide 1 to 1 1/2 lbs. grain per day per 100 lbs. of body weight. Offer a loose salt-mineral mix free choice.

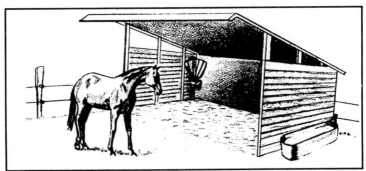

CHECK WITH YOUR VETERINARIAN. Before you start using a herd health program such as this one, discuss how it will fit your particular situation with your own veterinarian.

October, November, December

Deworm.

Evaluate open mares. Palpate and use ultrasound, culture, biopsy and caslicks as required.

Provide Tetanus Toxoid boosters as needed.

Evaluate young horses for muscle and skeletal development.

Chapter 56

Modern Concepts Of Poultry Disease Control

A NUMBER OF years ago, diseases such as pullorum, paratyphoid and fowl typhoid were a real problem to the hatcheryman and poultry producer. Many flocks had to be destroyed at a young age when they were found infected with pullorum or typhoid.

The discovery that these diseases were egg-transmitted and their presence in a breeder flock could be detected by a testing procedure was instrumental in bringing about the low incidence or pullorum and typhoid now found in poultry flocks.

At one time, paratyphoid was also a serious problem to the turkey industry. This has been virtually eliminated as a result of the Salmonella typhymurium control programs now in effect. More recently infectious sinusitis (Mycoplasma gallisepticum infection) has been reduced to a low incidence in turkey flocks as a result of testing turkey breeder flocks for this disease.

Coccidiosis and blackhead, two diseases that were real problems in earlier years, can now be effectively controlled by use of preventive medications in the feed.

Vaccines Are The Real Key

The discovery of vaccines to prevent Newcastle disease, infectious bronchitis, avian encephalomyelitis, laryngotracheitis, fowl pox and Marek's disease have eliminated many disease hazards of poultry production. Without these vaccines it would be impossible to raise birds in the large multiple confinement units such as we have today.

Coronaviral enteritis of turkey (bluecomb), a disease that earlier appeared continuously on turkey farms causing serious losses, can now be controlled by depopulation and security programs. Turkeys recovering from coronaviral infection are immune for life, although they may continue to be carriers and shedders of the virus. The controlled depopulation of turkeys on farms and in areas where this disease exists, along with a proper security program, is the only way to eliminate the disease. This approach has been used with a high degree of success in areas that previously experienced problems controlling this infection.

Diseases Are Still A Concern

With disease control testing programs plus numerous vaccines and drugs available for preventing poultry diseases, raising poultry free of disease might appear to be an easy goal to attain. However, this is not the case.

New diseases are emerging all the time and old diseases have been waiting for an opportunity to again obtain a foothold in poultry flocks. Infectious coryza, a disease that once was practically nonex-

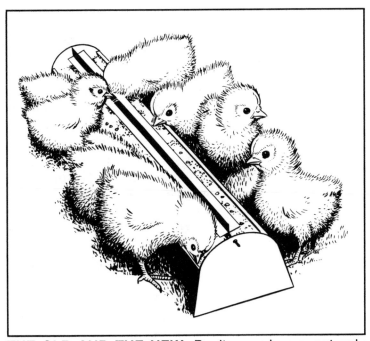

THE OLD AND THE NEW. Poultry producers not only have to be on the lookout for many new disease problems, but some of the older diseases which have not proven troublesome for some time are now making a comeback.

istent, has again made its appearance in large laying complexes. Mycoplasma gallisepticum (CRD) is a serious problem in large laying units. These two diseases will remain in a building continuously unless there is an all-in all-out program.

Fowl cholera, another old disease, has become a real hazard to the turkey industry in areas of high density. The development of resistant strains of the organism to numerous medications that were effective in controlling the disease has made it one of the more alarming diseases in the industry. Further research is needed to develop an immunizing product that will induce immunity against all strains of the organism.

Confinement Brought New Pressures

Colibacillosis, coli-septecemia, or E. coli infection, caused by Escherichia coli is another old disease making an unfortunate comeback. It was not of much importance until chickens and turkeys were raised in large confinement units and multiple brooding was practiced. Unfortunately, floor-pen production practices present ideal conditions for this organism to reproduce and concentrate large numbers of the organism in a small area.

There are also other factors which allow certain strains of E. coli to assume disease-producing capabilities. Environmental factors in a building such as chilling, overcrowding, wet, humid and unsanitary conditions are factors that can contribute to outbreaks of this disease. Other diseases such as mycoplasmosis, viral diseases, coccidiosis and other diseases capable of stressing the flock may also lead to E. coli outbreaks. Once the disease establishes itself in a flock, it is difficult to control because of the organism's resistance to most drugs.

New Diseases Coming

In addition to a number of old diseases that are re-emerging, some new diseases are being seen for the first time. As an example, poultry pathologists have described new strains of bronchitis and eight strains of adenovirus. Inclusion bursal disease (Gumboro disease), viral arthritis and other new viruses will continue to be discovered as causes of economic losses in poultry production.

Modern pullet growing management is resulting in 20-week-old pullets which have little experience dealing with mild disease agents. Breeders who have eliminated Mycoplasma gallisepticum and Mycoplasma synoviae from their flocks normally maintain a very tight security program. This has resulted in the elimination of exposure of the pullet to some microorganisms previously felt to be non-pathogenic. New housing systems have enabled producers to grow tens of thousands of pullets off the floor in new housing with no exposure to "normal" chicken viruses.

Replacement pullets, with little immunity to any of the "normal" microorganisms, may encounter an environment loaded with these agents. These encounters with unfamiliar agents often cause new diseases that have never before observed by poultry pathologists. Exposure to these new agents by pullets coming into production undoubtedly influences their productivity throughout the laying cycle. The greatest disease exposure normally occurs in multiple age farms.

New Approaches To Disease Control

Bacterial and viral diseases can be prevented by following several different approaches.

One method is to eliminate the pathogen. This procedure has been successful against Mycoplasma gallisepticum and coryza. It has been partially successful against laryngotracheitis and several other diseases.

Another method of control of poultry diseases can help in reducing the number of pathogens. This has been proven very successful by using strict sanitation measures against pathogens such as E. coli and Marek's disease.

The third idea is to increase the resistance of the host. This procedure is accomplished by vaccination which has been very successful against diseases such as Newcastle, Marek's disease, laryngotracheitis and others.

Colibacillosis, fowl cholera and arthritis continue to be problems in turkey flocks. Hemorrhagic enteritis and ulcerative enteritis present problems in certain areas.

More Research Is Needed

The chicken is the domestic animal which has the greatest number of infectious diseases. Tremendous strides have been made in controlling these diseases. However, much more remains to be done if the poultry industry is to continue to expand. As a result, there will be a tremendous demand for improved vaccines, improved methods of vaccine testing, improved immunization programs and improved methods of disease control and eradication.

Chapter 57

Poultry Disease Management For Peak Egg Production

THE FOLLOWING provides a brief rundown on critical disease management ideas for laying hens.

Chicks

Young birds require plenty very special attention.

Coccidiosis

Prevention: Use a coccidiostat which is recommended by your veterinarian.

Treatment: Furazolidone at 0.011% for 5 to 7 days.

Drug Withholding Period: 5 days.

Salmonella Pullorum

Prevention: Obtain chicks from a pullorum-free source. Add 0.011% of Furazolidone for 2 weeks.

Treatment: Feed Furazolidone at 0.011% in feed.

Drug Withholding Period: 5 days.

Chronic Respiratory Disease

This disease is also known as Mycoplasma gallisepticum.

Prevention: Obtain chicks from a clean source.

Treatment: Feed Chlortetracycline at 100 to 200 grams per ton.

Colibacillosis E. Coli

Prevention: Feed Sulfadimethoxine at a rate of 0.0125%.

Treatment: Feed Oxytetracycline at a rate of 100 to 200 grams per ton.

Drug Withholding Period: 3 to 5 days, depending on which drug is used.

Fowl Typhoid

Prevention: Add Furazolidone at 0.011% for 14 days in feed.

Treatment: Add Furazolidone at a rate of 0.011% in feed for 2 weeks.

Drug Withholding Period: 5 days.

Laryngotracheitis Virus

Prevention: Live virus vaccine.

Treatment: None.

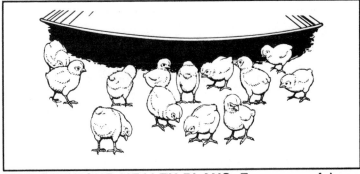

MAP OUT YOUR HEALTH PLANS. For successful egg production, you need to have separate detailed health plans for both your young chicks and your flock of pullets.

Infectious Bronchitis

Prevention: Live virus vaccine.

Treatment: None.

Fowl Pox Virus

Prevention: Vaccine.

Treatment: None.

Newcastle Disease Virus

Prevention: Vaccine.

Treatment: None.

Marek's Disease

Prevention: Vaccinate at 1 day of age.

Treatment: None.

Pullets

A successful egg producing program will also zero in on the control of a number of potentially-costly diseases that can not only reduce production but also result in unnecessary death losses.

Chronic Respiratory Disease

Prevention: Use a killed bacterin or live vaccine.

Treatment: Feed Tylosin at a rate of 1,000 grams per ton.

Drug Withholding Period: 5 days.

Fowl Cholera

Prevention: Killed bacterin.

Treatment: Use Sulfadimethoxine at a rate of 0.05% per gallon of water for 5 to 7 days.

Drug Withholding Period: 5 days.

Coryza

Prevention: Killed bacterin. Feed Erythromycin at a rate of 92.5 grams per ton for 10 days.

Treatment: Feed Erythromycin at a rate of 185 grams per ton for 5 to 8 days. Or mix it at a rate of 2 grams in each 5 gal. of water.

Drug Withholding Period: 2 days.

Chapter 58

Respiratory Diseases Of Laying Hens

THE RESPIRATORY diseases found in layers are generally caused by virus, mycoplasma and bacterial agents.

Major Disease Causing Agents

Most respirary problems are caused by one or more of the following:

Viral Respiratory Diseases

- Newcastle disease (ND).

- Infectious bronchitis (IB).

- Laryngotracheitis (LT).

- Fowl pox (FP), wet form.

- Adenovirus.

All of these viral diseases, except for adenovirus, can be controlled through proper vaccination. Vaccinating for fowl pox and laryngotracheitis should be used only if there is a problem on your farm or in your geographical area.

Mycoplasma Diseases

- M. gallisepticum (MG).

- M. synoviae (MS).

M. gallisepticum and M. synoviae are best controlled by eradication of these diseases in breeder herds and by practicing a good preventive program for pullets and hens.

Bacterial Respiratory Diseases

- Infectious coryza.

- Localized pasteurellosis.

Both coryza and fowl cholera are best controlled by preventing their introduction onto your farm. These two diseases remain endemic on infected premises. Complete depopulation is recommended on farms which have experienced these two diseases.

Typical Disease Symptoms

Newcastle Disease: This disease has a sudden onset accompanied by acute respiratory signs, production drop and possible development of some nervous signs.

Infectious Bronchitis: It is recognized by a sudden onset, severe respiratory symptoms and a precipitous drop in egg production.

Laryngotracheitis: This disease has a sudden to gradual onset, causes moderate drop in production, labored breathing, gasping and an occasional high-pitched stress sound.

Fowl pox (Wet Form): It causes labored breathing in the birds with lesions in the throat. Lesions of pox can be observed on some birds.

Infectious Coryza: It causes facial swelling, clear amber stick fetid nasal exudate and a drop in production.

M. Gallisepticum And M. Synoviae: They cause mild respiratory symptoms, nasal exudate and a moderate drop in production.

Adenovirus: It produces a very mild respiratory reaction, a mild drop in egg production which may be accompanied by egg deformity and a drop in the percentage of grade "A" eggs being produced.

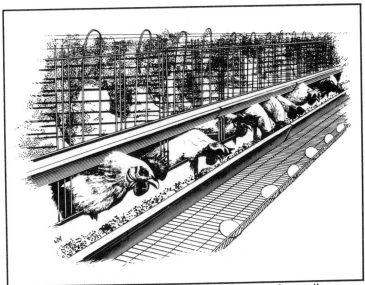

START EARLY IN LIFE. The control of various diseases with a vaccination program must start during the grow-out period for replacement pullets. It must also continue in the laying house, being carried out throughout each hen's life.

Treatment Recommendations

Medications are normally administered with respiratory diseases in layers, but there is no guarantee as to their benefit. Flock management and treatment during disease outbreaks basically centers around good nursing, increased security, correcting environmental errors and the administration of medications when indicated.

Treatment recommendations include:

Newcastle Disease, Infectious Bronchitis: There is no treatment that is specific, but broad spectrum antibiotics may be used.

Laryngotracheitis, Fowl pox: Antibiotics, particularly tylosin, erythromycin and tetracyclines are normally used with outbreaks of these diseases.

Fowl Cholera And Coryza: Use sulfas and antibiotics.

Adenovirus: Use antibiotics and vitamin fortification.

Vaccination Schedule

The control of diseases by vaccination must start during the growing period of the replacement pullets, then continue in the laying house throughout the life of the hens. Vaccines must be handled properly, administered correctly and a definite program followed if the immunization program is to be successful.

1 Day

Vaccine: Marek's.

Method Of Application: Subcutaneously.

10 to 14 Days

Vaccine: Newcastle B1 or La Sota.

Method Of Application: Individual bird application with Intraocular or intranasal methods.

4 to 5 Weeks

Vaccine: La Sota. Vaccinate again with La Sota at 12 to 14 weeks and every 60 days thereafter.

Method Of Application: Use either individual (intraocular or intranasal) or mass (spray or in water) treatments.

6 to 20 Weeks

Vaccine: Laryngotracheitis.

Method Of Application: Vent-brush vaccine or eye-drop vaccine.

8 to 16 Weeks

Vaccine: Fowl pox.

Method Of Application: Wing-web or feather follicle.

10 to 16 Weeks

Vaccine: Epidemic tremors.

Method Of Application: Live virus vaccine, water or a killed virus vaccine administered at 15 to 20 weeks.

12 to 18 Weeks

Vaccine: Bronchitis.

Method Of Application: Apply in water, intraocular or intranasal.

Chapter 59

Handling Turkey Disease Problems

REGARDLESS OF how many birds you happen to raise, there are seven major types of diseases you need to be on the lookout for with turkeys.

E. Coli Infection

The severity of this disease varies from minor death losses up to where 50% of the flock can be lost during the first 8 weeks of life. Many outbreaks are caused by a combination of agents that can further stress the flock, resulting in a higher death loss than when E. coli alone was involved. E. coli is also frequently isolated in conjunction with other diseases. This further complicates the disease syndrome and makes it more difficult to get a response from any prescribed treatment.

More information is definitely needed about E. coli infection, such as the sources of pathogenic serotypes of E. coli, how E. coli is introduced into the turkey flock, how it can be prevented and how it can best be treated. A great deal more research will be necessary before these questions can be answered.

The treatment of E. coli infection in turkeys has often proven very disappointing. It requires management programs at every level of production to minimize the buildup of E. coli in a turkey house environment. Other diseases occurring concurrently with colibacillosis and further complicating the disease and exaggerating death losses are mycoplasma infections, unknown viral respiratory disease agents, Newcastle disease and coccidiosis.

Respiratory Diseases

Unfortunately, the causes of all respiratory disease symptoms in turkeys aren't fully known. However, it has become difficult to raise a flock of turkeys without some signs of respiratory disease developing.

The problems usually include nasal discharge, eye discharge, sneezing and coughing. These symptoms frequently appear during the first 5 weeks of life. The cause of these symptoms can't always be determined. Due to the additional stress produced by respiratory disease, the turkey flock also becomes more susceptible to other diseases such as colibacillosis.

Fowl Cholera

Fowl cholera can be found in most turkey raising situations. And, the judicious use of the best bacterins has failed to prevent heavy losses on many farms. Medication seems to become less and less effective.

In 1970, an isolate of the fowl cholera organism was discovered at Clemson Univ. which had low virulence and was capable of immunizing turkeys when administered in drinking water. This vaccine, known as CU oral fowl cholera vaccine, made it possible for a number of large-scale growers to continue in turkey production.

Growers should be aware that this oral vaccine will protect birds against all known strains of fowl cholera when used properly. This is a live vaccine that must be used exactly as prescribed.

Leg Problems

Leg weakness has long been recognized as a major economic problem in the turkey industry. Despite a great deal of research on leg weakness in turkey poults, no immediate practical controls have been developed to limit the disease in commercial flocks. Leg problems in turkey flocks in some areas often

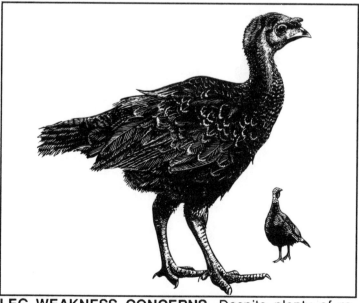

LEG WEAKNESS CONCERNS. Despite plenty of research on leg weakness in turkey poults, there are no practical vaccinations or medications which can be used to limit the losses due to this disease in commercial flocks.

413

present a serious problem while other areas experience very little incidence. Leg weakness has been known to occur on the same farm year-after-year.

Certain organisms are involved in leg weakness in turkey flocks. These include mycoplasma, staphylococci, E. coli, streptococci and the salmonellas. Other organisms can also be isolated from leg joints associated with specific diseases such as erysipelas and fowl cholera.

Generally speaking, treatment of leg problems in turkeys has been very discouraging. Each flock has to be evaluated separately and a determination made as to the particular problem.

Salmonella, Arizona Infections

Because salmonella and Arizona infections are widespread in turkeys, many hatcheries inject day-old poults with an antibiotic. While it has helped minimize losses from these infections, this type of treatment has not controlled the incidence of these infections.

If headway is to be made in controlling salmonella infections, special attention has to be given to providing salmonella-free feed ingredients, maintaining a salmonella-free environment and maintaining salmonella-and Arizona-free breeding flocks.

Aspergillosis

This disease, essentially involved with the respiratory system, is caused by a mold. Birds affected with this mold usually have difficulty breathing. Gasping, accelerated breathing and signs of nervous involvement are often observed in infected flocks.

This disease is generally seen in young birds as a result of contaminated litter, brooder houses and brooding equipment. Since most flocks are now grown under confinement conditions, the disease has become more prevalent. A house contaminated with this mold has to be thoroughly cleaned and disinfected before it is safe for turkeys.

There is no effective treatment for birds infected with aspergillosis.

Erysipelas

This is a highly infectious disease of turkeys. The incidence is much higher in tom flocks than hen flocks. This is probably due to the fighting activities of toms which spread the disease through skin abrasions rather than the tom simply being more susceptible to this problem.

The disease occurs every year on some farms. Most outbreaks occur in semi-adult and adult birds prior to marketing age. Since erysipelas is difficult to control by medication, there is a constant "above average" death loss.

Poultry farms experiencing this disease should

consider a vaccination program which can be effective in controlling death loss.

Disease Prevention Programs

In order to survive in the turkey industry, losses from disease have to be minimized. This doesn't happen without considerable thought and planning. A preventive health program must be planned well in advance of the next growing season. Effective vaccination programs are available for fowl cholera, erysipelas, Newcastle disease, fowl pox and avian encephalomyelitis.

Diseases such as coccidiosis and blackhead are effectively prevented through medication pro-

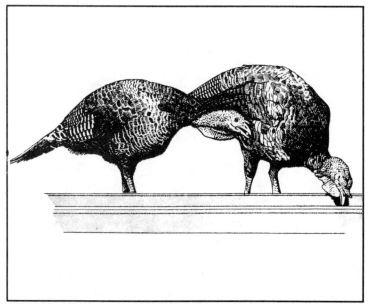

PREVENTIVE HEALTH PLANS WORK. Map out health management programs well before your turkey poults arrive. Losses can be sharply reduced if you and your veterinarian put together a health plan that will really work.

grams. Crop mycosis is another disease which can be effectively prevented with drugs.

One of the hardest programs to sell to a turkey grower is the prevention of disease problems through good management. It is too easy for a turkey producer to hope that his defective management procedures may be overcome by the addition of a few drugs or antibiotics in the feed or water.

Instead, you need to realize that having an effective management program requires the rigid enforcement of a number of basic health rules.

Disease Sources

There are three general sources of disease problems found with turkeys:

The Environment On The Farm

Harmful microorganisms and parasites may survive in the turkey house in litter or dust. Buildings may be such that they can't be thoroughly cleaned and disinfected, thus there is no easy way to decontaminate a building. A number of organisms such as salmonellas, Arizona paracolons and coliforms can survive for weeks or months in the dust, litter or soil found in the turkey house.

Infection From Outside The Farm

Control over the introduction of harmful diseases onto the turkey farm basically rests with the complex's managers. The proper control of traffic onto the farm (such as visitors, processing trucks, feed trucks, poultry equipment, etc.) is very important to reducing the potential for disease outbreaks.

It is the job of you as a manager to determine what your policy will be and then to set up and enforce guidelines to minimize the possible introduction of costly disease problems.

Infection Carrier, Reservoirs On The Farm

Some bacteria or viruses may survive many months or even from one year to the next in the living host. As an example, turkeys surviving an outbreak of fowl cholera will remain carriers of the organisms and serve as a serious source of infection for other flocks.

Turkeys surviving an outbreak of bluecomb disease are carriers. They will perpetuate the disease if carried over from one year to the next in breeder flocks. Free-flying birds on a farm may also carry such diseases as salmonellosis, fowl cholera, mycoplasmosis, Newcastle disease and many other diseases.

Appendix A

Know What These Words Mean

Use this handy reference guide to review many of the various animal health terms which are were used throughout this book. A number of additional important animal health terms for the layman are definied in Appendix B.

 A

Abscess. A localized collection of pus in a cavity formed by the disintegration of tissue.

Acute. Sharp, having a short and rather severe course.

Aerobe. A micro-organism which can live and grow in the presence of free oxygen.

Anaphylaxis. An unusual or exaggerated reaction of the organism to foreign protein or other substances.

Anemia. A condition in which the blood is deficient in quality or quantity. Can be local or general.

Anthelmintic. Destructive to worms.

Antibiotic. Destructive to life. A chemical substance produced by micro-organisms which has the capacity, in dilute solutions, to inhibit the growth of, or to destroy, bacteria and other micro-organisms.

Antibody. A modified serum globulin synthesized by an animal in response to antigenic stimulus, which reacts specifically in the animal and in laboratory equipment with the homologous antigen.

Antidote. A substance to counteract a poison.

Antigen. A high-molecular-weight substance or complex, usually protein or protein-polysaccharide in nature. When foreign to the blood-stream, on gaining access to the tissue of an animal, it will stimulate the formation of a specific antibody and react specifically with it.

Antiseptic. A substance which will inhibit growth and development of micro-organisms without necessarily destroying them.

Antiserum. A serum that contains antibodies which usually results from the hyperimmunization against one or more infectious agents.

Antitoxin. Antibody to the toxin of a micro-organism, usually the bacterial exotoxins that combine specifically with the toxin with neutralization of the toxicity.

Atrophy. A defect or failure of nutrition of a tissue or organ manifest as a wasting away of a cell, tissue, organ or parts.

Attenuate. To render less virulent.

Avirulent. Not disease producing.

 B

Bactericidal. Capable of destroying bacteria.

Bacterin. A vaccine of bacterial growth.

Bacteriostatic. Inhibits bacterial growth.

Biological. Referring to life or vaccine, bacterin or antiserum type product.

Blood Serum. The clear liquid which separates from the blood when it clots; therefore, blood plasma from which fibrinogen has been removed.

 C

Catarrh. Inflammation of a mucous membrane.

Cell. Any one of the minute protoplasmic masses which make up organized tissue—circumscribed mass of protoplasm containing a nucleus in most instances.

Chronic. Long, lengthy, continued.

Colostrum. The fluid secreted by the mammary gland a few days before and after parturition.

Conjunctivitis. Inflammation of the delicate membrane that lines the eyelids and eyeball.

Contagious. Capable of being transmitted from one to another.

 E

Edema. The presence of abnormally large amounts of fluid in the intercellular spaces.

Emetic. A medicine that causes vomiting.

Encephalitis. Inflammation of the brain.

Endemic. Restricted to a reasonably small geographical area in the animal.

Endotoxin. A toxic substance formed within the bacterial cell.

Enteric. Pertaining to the small intestine.

Enteritis. Inflammation of the small intestine.

Epithelium. The covering of the internal and external surfaces of the body.

Erythrocyte. "Red" blood cell—a circular biconcave disc, containing hemoglobin found in the blood.

Etiology. The study or theory of the causation of any disease.

Expectorant. A medicine which aids in expulsion of mucous and exudate from the lungs.

Exudate. A substance which is deposited in or on animal tissue by a vital process or disease.

 F

Febrile. Having an elevated body temperature.

 G

Globulin. A class of proteins insoluble in water but soluble in saline solution or water soluble proteins. (Antibodies are mostly gamma globulins).

Gram negative. Losing the stain or decolorized by alcohol in Grams' method of staining (rose colored).

Gram positive. Retaining the stain and resisting decolorization by alcohol in Grams' method of staining (purple colored).

Hematoma. An enlarged area containing effused blood.

Hemoglobin. The oxygen-carrying red pigment of the red blood corpuscle. It is a reddish crystalizable conjugated protein consisting of the protein "globin" combined with the prosthetic "heme."

Hepatitis. Inflammation of the liver. The morbid enlargement or over-growth of an organ or part due to an increase in size of its constituent cells.

Hyper-immune. To repeatedly expose an animal with an antigen so as to produce a large quantity of antibodies as in production of an antiserum.

Icterus. Jaundice, yellowish color in tissues.

Immunity. Represents protection against any particular disease or poison.

Infection. Invasion of the body by pathogenic micro-organisms and the reaction of the tissues to their presence and the toxins generated by them.

Inflammation. The condition into which tissues enter as a reaction to injury by trauma or toxins.

Inoculate. To introduce immune serum, vaccine bacterin, toxoid or live micro-organisms on to a medium for their reproduction.

Intramuscular. Into the muscle.

Intraperitoneal. Between the two layers of peritoneum in the abdominal cavity.

Intravenous. Within the vein.

Keratoconjunctivitis. Inflammation of the cornea and conjunctiva (membranes of the eye).

L

Leukocyte. White blood cell. There are several types.

Leukocytosis. An abnormal decrease in the amount of white blood cells.

Lysis. Destruction of cells or other substances by dissolving.

 M

Malignant. Tending to go from bad to worse; capable of spreading or enlarging.

Mastitis. Inflammation of the mammary gland or glands.

Metritis. Inflammation of the uterus.

Milli. A prefix denoting one-thousandth part.

Modified live virus. Usually refers to a virus that has been intentionally changed to be safe for use as a vaccine with tissue cell culture.

Mucous membrane. Epethelial cells found upon a basement membrane—lining the canals and cavities of the body that communicate with external air.

Mucus. The free slime of mucous membranes.

Mycosis. Any disease caused by a fungus.

Mycotoxin. A fungal or bacterial toxin.

 N

Necrosis. Death of a cell or group of cells which is in contact with living tissue.

Necropsy. An examination after death usually involving some dissection of the animal.

Neonatal. Pertaining to the first part of life.

Nephritis. Inflammation of the kidney.

Neurotoxin. A substance that is poisonous or destructive to nerve tissue.

Node (lymph). A gland-like structure in the lymphatic system that filters and produces blood constituents.

O

Oncogenic. Giving rise to tumors or causing tumor formation; especially of viruses inducing tumors.

Orchitis. Inflammation of a testicle.

Osmosis. The passage of a pure solvent from the lesser to the greater concentration when two solutions are separated by a membrane which selectively prevents the passage of solute molecules, but is permeable to the solvent.

Otitis. Inflammation of the ear.

 P

Pathogen. Any disease-producing micro-organism.

Pathogenic. Giving origin to disease.

Peritoneum. The serous membrane lining the abdominal walls and viscera.

Pleura. The membrane covering the lungs and lining the chest cavity.

Prophylaxis. The prevention of disease.

Pulmonary. Pertaining to the lungs.

Purulent. Consisting of or containing pus.

Pus. A liquid inflammation material made up of white blood cells.

 R

Rhinitis. Inflammation of the mucous membrane of the nose— degenerative disease of turbinate (nasal) bones in swine.

 S

Sanguinous. Pertaining to blood.

Septicemia. Micro-organisms with their toxins in the blood and, therefore, throughout the animal.

Serum. the clear portion of any animal liquid separated from its more solid elements—especially the liquid which separates from the clot and corpuscles of blood.

Shock. A condition of acute peripheral circulatory failure due to derangement of circulatory control or loss of circulating fluid.

Somatic. Pertaining to the body.

Stable cell line. A type of selected cells for tissue culture purposes, the properties of which are known, do not contribute variances and contaminants to vaccines produced with them.

Stomatitis. Inflammation of the membranes of the mouth.

Subclinical. Without obvious symptoms, but still diseased.

Subcutaneous. Under the skin.

 T

Tissue cell culture. Growth of live cells, usually of animal origin, in laboratory ware for production of modified live viral vaccines.

Thrombosis. A blood clot in a vessel or cavity which remains in place.

Titer. The quantity of a substance required to produce a reaction with a given volume of another substance.

Toxemia. Toxins in the blood of an animal.

Toxin. Any poisonous substance.

Toxoid. A "decay" product of bacterial toxins that has lost its toxicity, but can stimulate anti-toxin formation.

Trachitis. Inflammation of the trachea.

 U

Uremia. The presence of urinary constituents in the bladder.

 V

Vaccine. A suspension of attenuated or killed micro-organisms used to stimulate antibodies when administered to a susceptible subject.

Vector. A carrier of disease from one animal to another (usually an arthropod).

Vesicle. A small sac or blister containing fluid.

Villi. Small vascular processes or protrusions growing on a mucous membrane as in the digestive system.

Viremia. Virus in the blood.

Virucidal. Capable of neutralizing or destroying a virus.

Virulence. The degree of pathogenecity or disease-producing potency of a micro-organism as indicated by its ability to invade the host or rate of fatality.

Viscera. Large internal organs of the body.

Commonly-Used Lay Terms

This reference contains definitions for a number of the commonly used animal health terms. Other frequently used health terms are defined in Appendix A.

 B

Blind teat. Atresia of teat canal or cistern.

Blow Out. Prolapsed rectum.

 C

Calf Jack. Fetal extractor.

Cast Her Whithers. Prolapsed uterus.

Cat. Tom or King = male.
Pussy or Queen = female.
Kitten = young.
Pride = group.

Cattle. Bull = male.
Cow = female.
Calf = young.
Steer = castrated male.
Heifer = young female.
Drove = herd on the move.

Cod. Fat filled scrotum.

Cow To Clean. Retained placenta.

Cribber. Animal biting or setting teeth against something and "sucking wind".

Critter. Semi-mature steer.

Cut. Castrate.

 D

Dog. Dog = male.
Bitch = female.
Pup = young.

 G

Geld. Castrate horse.

Goat. Billy or Buck = male.
Nanny or Doe = female.
Kid = young.

Gomer. Sterile teaser bull.

L

Line Back. Stripe backed animal (usually Hereford).

 P

Pick Their Pockets. Castration.

Pig. Boar = male.
Sow = female.
Pig or Shoat = young.
Gilt = nonparous female.
Hog = large pig.
Barrow = castrated male.

Plastic Bull. Artificial inseminator.

Pull A Calf. Calf delivery.

 R

Roan. Mixture of white and color in hair coat.

 S

Slab Sided. Thin; can count ribs.

Smooth Mouth. Aged horse or cow.

Snorter. Excitable animal.

Spaded or Spay. Ovariohysterectomy.

Spook. Nervous horse or cow.

Springer. Heifer about to calve.

Stag. Male castrated late in life.

Stocking-Up. Swollen legs.

Stud. Stallion; or male dog.

Sugar Eater. Pampered animal.

Sulfur. Sulfa drugs.

Swamp Angels Or Hillbillies. Inferior cattle.

 T

Threw Her Calf Bed. Prolapsed uterus.

Tie. Area of hide adhering to vertebrae, a dimple like depression.

Tube A Horse. Nasal-gastric tube insertion.

Tucked Up. Drawn up in flanks.

 W

Wattle. Owner mark on neck or jaw made by cutting loose skin.

Index

Where To Find What You Need

Rely on this easy-to-use alphabetical index to find detailed information on all livestock health topics found in this book.

D

 E

688480